# Good Health through Grains

## Regina Nedas

0

Editor: Philip L. Levin, MD

Published by Doctor's Dreams Publishing
PO Box 4808
Biloxi, MS  39535
www.Doctors-Dreams.com
writerpllevin@gmail.com

Prepared in the United States of America

ISBN:  978-1-942181-30-9

# Good Health through Grains

# Regina Nedas

**A discussion of the nutritional value of various grains including recipes.**

# Table of Contents

Page

## NOTE TO THE READER

This book is not meant to offer medical advice or prescriptions. It does not provide a cure for diseases but rather a diet that helps improve health and prevent disease. Certain therapies will work better for some people than for others. Some gluten free grains interact with prescribed medications, or cause allergic reactions, such as rashes, itching, or bloating. We recommend that any medical issues be discussed with a qualified nutritionist or health care professional. If you are taking prescription medications, do not quit taking them to try a replacement from the book without consulting your physician.

## PREFACE

Hippocrates said: "Food is your medicine, and medicine is your food." This saying is as relevant today as it was two thousand years ago.

I lived in Europe for many years where I was a university instructor in botany and microbiology. There I developed my interest in the medicinal use of plants and grains, studying their healing benefits in the human body. In my travels across Europe and Asia, I've collected recommendations from around the world about healthy lifestyles, ethnic medicine, and natural curative techniques. This book includes folk and ethnic medicine from Lithuania, Russia, The Caucasus, China, Tibet, Egypt, India, Pakistan, and North America. From each area I interviewed natives and studied old texts to acquire information about local medicinal herbs and grains, much of it unique and ancient. I have integrated this information with modern scientific knowledge.

This book only briefly touches on the main topic of food and health. For much more extensive information, please consult my two-hundred-page book *The Therapy Of Natural Living*, complete with over 100 recipes, available through Amazon in soft color or as an e-book.

# INTRODUCTION

*"The mind is the greatest gift of nature. It elevates us above our passions and shortcomings and helps us make proper use of our strengths, talents, and virtues." –* Nicholas Sebastian de Samfore.

Our ancestors successfully used natural medicinal plants and grains for their health needs. In ancient times, people harnessed the power of healing herbs, plants, fruits, grains, and oils to aid their life expectancy, strength, endurance, working capacity, ability to work, and energy levels.

This book provides a guide to those gluten free grains and their uses. I have drawn over thirty years of research and use of natural remedies to describe the use of natural products for health benefits.

*"Medicus-Curat, Natura-sanat."* Medicine Protects, Nature Heals – St. Hildegard von Bingen. 1098-1179. CAUSAE ET CURAE.

## WHAT WE LEARN FROM OUR DISEASES

*"It would not be good if all our desires were fulfilled: only when we become ill do we understand what kind of wealth is health, only having experienced evil do we appreciate the goodness, only when we are hungry do we feel the taste of meal, only when we get tired do we enjoy our rest".* – Hersclitus, Greek philosopher, 535 BC-475 BC.

In order to stay healthy or to recover faster from illnesses, it is important to bear a few things in mind; namely, to enjoy every moment of our lives, love yourself and others sincerely, laugh, and have as much fun as possible. It is important to learn from our experiences and get rid of erratic stereotypes.
Create a new standard of living for yourself and strive for the best health.
Live a long life without losing vigor.

REFLECTIONS
The best foods are those that give health.
The greatest mind is God.
The greatest sin is fear.
The best day is today.
The best job is the one you love.
The greatest weakness is hatred.
The most dangerous man is a liar.
The greatest need is communication.
The greatest asset is health.
The greatest gift you can give or receive is love.
Man's greatest friend is a good book.
Your enemies are jealousy, greed, indulgence, and self-pity.
The greatest fullness of life is physical, mental, and spiritual perfection.
The most repulsive trait is cruelty.
The most unpleasant feature is bloat.
The biggest obstacle is sadness.
The most intelligent person is the one who is able to realize his accomplishments.

## FAVORITE SAYINGS ABOUT HEALTH AND WELLNESS

*Health is real wealth and not pieces of gold or silver.* – Mahatma Gandhi – 20th century philosopher

*The doctor of the future will no longer treat the human frame with drugs but rather will cure and prevent diseases with nutrition.* – Thomas Edison – 19th and 20th century inventor

*Health is a state of the body. Wellness is a state of being.* – Miles J. Stanford – 20th century Christian author

*The key to a healthy life is having a healthy mind.* – Richard Davidson – professor of psychology

*To keep the body in good health is a duty, otherwise we shall not be able to keep our mind strong and clear.* – Buddha – 6th century B.C. philosopher

*Health is like money. We never have a true idea of its value until we lose it.* – Josh Billings – 19th century American humorist

*A healthy outside starts from the inside.* – Robert Urich – actor

*The good deeds you do now are the treasures for the future.* – Philippine proverb

*Six things needed are a book, a clock, a shell, wisdom, the heart, and the imagination.* – Judy Kane

*Time and health are two precious assets that we don't recognize and appreciate until they have been depleted.* – Denis Waitley – 21st century motivational speaker

*The Lord has created medicines out of the earth, and he that is wise will not abhor them.* – King James Version, Ecclesiasticus 38:4

## 10 WAYS TO GOOD HEALTH

Less alcohol, more tea,
Less processed, more fresh,
Less meat, more vegetables,
Less sugar, more fruit,
Less eating, more chewing,
Less words, more action,
Less greed, more giving,
Less worry, more sleep,
Less driving, more walking,
Less anger, more laughter.

HEALTH OPPORTUNITIES TO IMPROVE YOUR
HEALTH AND LIFE

Eat a daily salad (leafy greens),
Adopt a daily tea habit (daytime green tea and
chamomile tea at bedtime),
Eat a daily banana (a diet rich in potassium),
Have a superberry dessert (dark-colored berries),
Use avocado instead of mayonnaise,
Drink your fiber (blend banana, orange, and spinach, and
throw in some walnuts),
Choose organic vegetables and fruits when possible,
Try natural laxatives (prunes, rhubarb, kiwi, linen seeds,
figs),
Avoid artificial sweets (aspartame, sucralose, saccharin,
neotame, and acesulfame potassium),
Check ingredients.
Bring plants into your house,
Avoid stress and anxiety,
Be a morning person,
Do an hourly posture check,
Make eye contact over dinner,
Do the boogie woogie (turn together nightly dance
party),
Give thanks after every meal, (this is a terrific habit),
Call one long-lost friend every week,
Give little gifts,
Once a week try something new (listen to new music,
learn some words in a foreign language, take dancing or
piano lessons.)
Stay active (go to for a walk, ride a bike),
Read a book,

Brush and floss regularly,
Do some art,
Portion out nuts,
Spend time in a nature (at least 20 minutes a day),
Store leftovers in glass containers instead of plastic,
Opt for fragrance-free products.

## A STORY OF TWO SEEDS

Two seeds lay side by side in the fertile autumn ground.

"I want to grow!" Said the first seed. "I want to root the roots and plant the seedlings. Welcoming spring, I want to unfold my delicate buds like flags. I long to feel the warmth of the sun on my face and the blessing of the morning dew on my petals!"

And it began to grow.

"What a fate!" the second seed murmured. "I'm afraid. If I let the roots go deep into the ground, I don't know what I will find there in the dark. If I sprout, hard clumps might injure my delicate sprouts. And if I unfold my buds, they can be cut by some snail. When I use my lovely petals, some child might pick me. No, I'd rather wait until it's safe enough."

And it waited.

In search of food, the hen crept into the yard. He saw the waiting seed and swallowed it.

It is important to take risks, for you never know your fate. Sometimes you'll succeed and sometimes you won't. But not taking risks guarantees failure.

Adopted from Bruno Ferrero

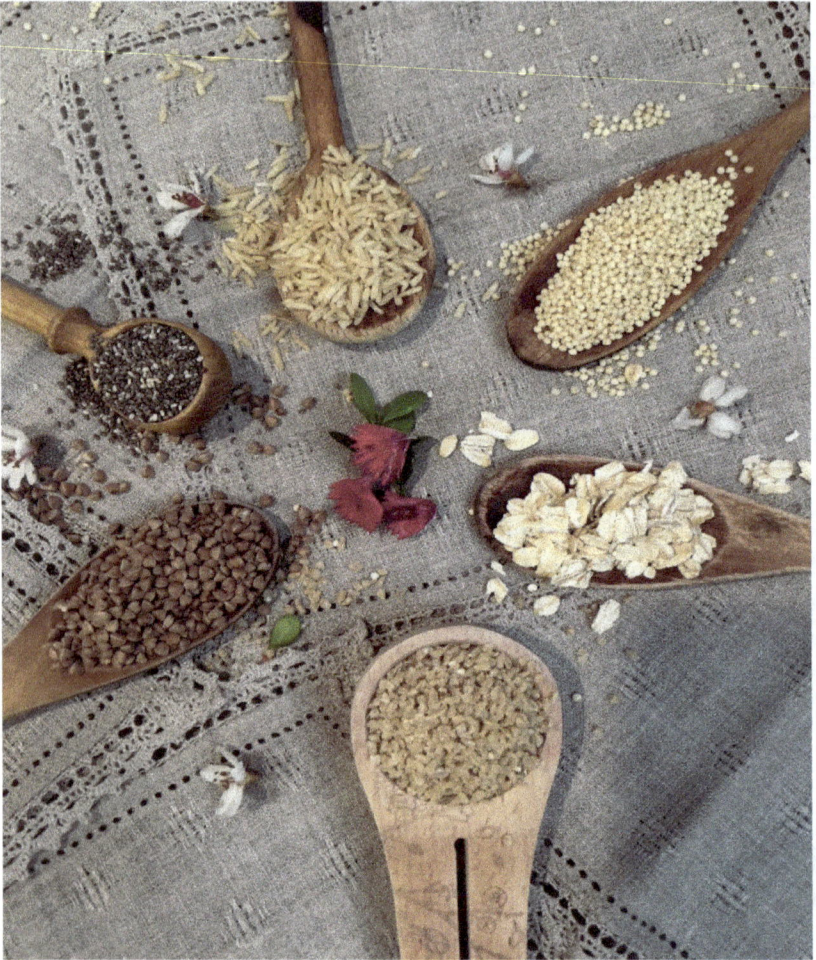

## Grains

*Look deep into nature, and then you will understand everything better.*
- Albert Einstein – Twentieth century physicist

Grains come from husked, crushed, or whole cereals, such as wheat, barley, buckwheat, oats, millet, quinoa, and rice. They are rich in carbohydrates (about 50-70%), thus making them a major source of energy. Grains also contain a considerable amount of protein. For example, oat grains have up to 15% protein, semolina 13%. They are also high in fat; oats contain about 8% fat and semolina about 1.4%. Grains provide vitamins B1, B2, PP, E, various minerals, and fiber.

**Ancient grains:** "Ancient grains" is a term used to describe a category of grains and cereals that have suffered only minimal changes over the millennia, only those changes used to sharpen their quality and yield. Ancient grains are more natural and more nutritious than those that have been genetically manipulated. Some are not necessarily grains - quinoa, for example, is actually a seed. Although they may seem new to Americans, ancient grains have long been popular in many parts of the world. Diets rich in these whole grains have been shown to be protective against chronic illness. They are high in fiber, vitamins, minerals, and proteins.

Recently, ancient grains are gaining popularity as more food importers provide the world with new foods to supply our ever-changing western palettes. Quinoa was the first ancient grain to grow in popularity, and others, like barley, were always around, but never particularly fashionable. Old or not, so-called ancient grains are all whole food grains, so for that reason they deserve attention as part of a healthy diet.

Ancient grains are not only "more natural," they also tend to be higher in fiber, protein, vitamins, and minerals. Ancient grains are often marketed as being more nutritious than modern grain, although their health benefits have been disputed by some nutritionists.

In contrast to ancient grains, most widespread cereals, including corn, rice, and modern varieties of wheat, are the products of recent crossbreeding and genetic manipulation. Modern wheat is grain that comes from a variety of wheat created in 1960. Not only has it undergone genetic tampering, but afterwards, the bleaching, stripping, and processing that modern wheat is subjected to during bread-making results in a very unnatural product. Modern wheat is high gluten with an increase in the protein parts that cause celiac disease, causing digestive problem, such as water retention, bloating, and gas.

Ancient grains can be used whole in pilafs, soups, salads, and stir-fry, or they can be soaked in flour and used for baking bread, pancakes, or just about in anything you would want to use flour. For example, Bulgarian's Boza is a malt drink made from millet flour.
Ancient grains include varieties of wheat. Spelt, einkorn, emmer, bulgur, barley, kamut, and farro are all members of the wheat family, and were eaten in medieval times. They are not gluten-free grains.

Spelt - high in protein and fiber.

Einkorn - domestic known as "petit epeautre" in French, Einkorn in German, or little spelt in England, "piccolo farro" in Italian and "escanda menor" in Spanish. High in protein, vitamins, minerals. Has a higher level of fat.

Emmer - has a special place in ancient Egypt where it was the main wheat cultivated in Pharaonic times. Emmer and barley were the primary ingredients in ancient Egypt used in making their bread and beer. Emmer was maybe one of the grains mentioned in ancient rabbinic texts as one of the five grains to be used by Jews during Passover for baking matzah. Emmer bread is available in the Netherlands and Switzerland. In parts of India, emmer wheat is grown as a drought and stress resistant wheat.

Bulgur - an expanding line of healthy grains. Bulgur is a staple food in many Mediterranean cultures. High in protein, fiber and minerals. Bulgur contains twice the fiber as oats, buckwheat or corn. Bulgur could be used as a replacement for rice in almost any recipe. It has a slightly nutty flavor to whatever it is combined with, making it a great compliment to almost any dish.

Barley - is a member of the grass family. It is self-pollinating. It has been used as animal fodder. Two-row barley is traditionally used in English ale-style beers. Six row barley is common in some American lager-style beers, especially when adjuncts such as corn and rice are used. Barley is an excellent source of fiber, manganese, selenium, and thiamine.

Kamut - has a nutty flavor and is high in fiber, protein and several minerals, including selenium and manganese. The firm texture and rich, nutty flavor make this heirloom grain a great addition to pilafs, soups, and cold salads.

Farro - type of grain with nutty flavor. High in Vitamin B3, fiber and nutrients. Hard to cook. It is likely to wind-up with teeth-breaking tough kernels. High in protein and fiber.

Ancient grains which are gluten free: millet, teff, oats, sorghum, quinoa, amaranth, buckwheat, and chia.

Millet - a small, whole grain is a staple in many Asian and African countries but thought of mostly as bird food in the United States. Millet is starchy, rich in protein.

Teff - common in Ethiopia, this grain has the highest calcium content.

Oats - rich in beta glucan. Protects the immune system against microbes and bacteria.

Sorghum - is a grass family Poaceae. Originally domesticated in Africa. When popped, it produces a product similar to popcorn, but the puffs are smaller. All sorghum contains phenolic acids and most contain flavonoids. Is correlated with antioxidant activity.

Quinoa - perhaps the best-known ancient grain. Quinoa has a great taste and nutritional properties. Quinoa is a one of nature's complete plant proteins, it has all nine essential amino acids in the right proportions to help support human nutritional needs.

Amaranth - a grain used by Aztecs, is both gluten-free and wheat-free and is a source of vitamin C.

Buckwheat - is a source of Vitamin B, nutrients, and minerals, high in potassium and iron.

Chia seeds - rich in Omega-3 fatty acids.

Brown rice - known as Asian rice. Great source of vitamins, minerals, fiber, and a good source of protein.

These alternative wheat products are healthier alternatives, more natural, and better for us, providing more vitamins, minerals, fiber, and protein than modern wheat-partly because they are rarely eaten in processed form.

"It has been a perfect storm for these ancient grains," says Cynthia Harriman, director of food and nutritional strategies at the non-profit organization, the Whole Grain Council. "They fit with our desire to look for super food, a magic bullet we should be eating."

Many of the grains are also gluten-free, or at least low in gluten, tapping into a growing demand from consumers.

"Part of the stories of these grains are the stories that surround them," says Harriman. "We are drawn to the idea that kamut comes from King Tutankhamun's tomb, the story draws our attention."

In BBC News Magazine' s Joanna Jolly asked, "Why do Americans love ancient grain?" Her answer: "It is a revolt against processed food. It is the opposite of modern."

*It is only the farmer who faithfully plants seeds in the*
*Spring, who reaps a harvest in the Autumn.*
--Bertie Charles Forbes, American author, founder
Forbes magazine, 1880-1954

**History:** The origin of grains goes back to the Neolithic
Revolution about 10,000 years ago, when prehistoric
communities started to make the transition from hunter -
gatherer to farmer. Ancient grains ranged across human
civilizations, from the Aztecs in the New World to the
Greeks and Egyptians in the old.

Quinoa, known as the "Mother Grain" in South
American culture, dates back to the Incan Empire and is
actually a seed not a grain. It was considered sacred by
the Inca people. Amaranth was likewise considered
sacred to the Aztecs, and was used as part of a religious
ceremony. To suppress their culture, the Spanish
colonial authorities banned its cultivation. Farro grains
are mentioned in the Old Testament.

Millet grains are mentioned in the Bible as an ingredient
for unleavened bread. Millet is one of the oldest foods
known to humans and possibly the first cereal grain to be
used for domestic purpose. Millet has been used in
Africa, China, and India as a staple food for thousands of
years and it was grown as early as 2700 BC in China. It
was documented that these millets were also grown by
lake dwellers of Switzerland during the Stone Age. In
time millets were spread throughout the world, The
Romans and Gauls made porridge with millet.

Commercial millet crops are produced by China, India, Greece, Egypt, and in parts of Africa.

Aztecs, Mayans, and other native American cultures valued chia seeds as a source of concentrated energy and nutrition. Chia means "Strength" in the Mayan's Language. Chia seeds served as a staple food for the Nahuatl (Aztec) cultures. Aztec warriors once used them for high energy endurance. This little super seed has survived through the ages and has become a valuable ingredient for gluten-free chefs.

Some say that Noah brought kamut kernels along on the ark, hence the nickname, "Prophet's wheat." Some claim kamut was found in the tomb of an Egyptian pharaoh.

Many of these grains have been planted and harvested in the same way for thousands of years.

By the end of the 19th century, grains were flushed with a hammer and then ground with handmade mills.

The first reference to ancient grains as a health food was in Daily News (New York) in 1996. Since then, the popularity of ancient grains as a food has increased and in 2011 the gluten-free food market was valued at $1.6 billion.

## The Six Most Popular Gluten-Free Grains

*I have the simplest of tastes. I am always satisfied with the best.*

- Oscar Wilde – 19th century poet and playwright

**Oats**. Oats (Avena sativa) is a species of cereal grain for its seeds. Sensitivity or allergy to oats is uncommon.

**Buckwheat.** Buckwheat (Fagopyrum esculentum) is not a type of wheat, as is not a grass. Instead buckwheat is related to sorrel, knotweed, and rhubarb. Buckwheat is referred to as pseudo cereal because its culinary use is the same as cereal. Buckwheat is a self-fertile plant This means it can self-produce, or in-breed, using its own pollen. Some people could be allergic to buckwheat.

**Quinoa**. Quinoa ( Chenopodium quinoa) is not a grass, but rather a pseudocereal related to spinach and amaranth (Amaranthus spp). It is a seed from vegetables. Belongs to the Amaranthaceae family. Young leaves are also nutritious and can be eaten as a vegetable botanically related to spinach, beets. Some people could be allergic to quinoa.

**Millet**. Millet (Paninium sumatrence) or bajra as it is called in Hindi is easily digestible and rarely causes any allergies.

**Brown Rice** (Ozyra sativa). It is a grass and belongs to the Poaceae family). When you have a wheat allergy, rice is a lifesaver and brown rice is particularly beneficial.

**Chia seeds**. Chia seeds (Salvia hispanica) are the edible seeds of a flowering plant in the mint family (Lamiaceae). Some people could be allergic to Chia seeds.

Be sure and check the packaging for a gluten-free declaration, as sometimes the manufacturer adds gluten containing products.

You need to soak chia seeds before cooking with them? Soaked chia seeds are easier to digest and absorb their nutrients. Soaking them causes a bit of sprouting, which releases the enzyme inhibitors that are used to protect the seed.

Soak chia seeds in 1 oz of seeds to10 oz of water and let them sit for between 30 minutes to two hours, or overnight.

Due to the presence of gluten in wheat, barley, and rye, the immune system of intolerant people may cause them to develop celiac disease. Celiac disease damages the small intestine and interferes with the absorption of nutrients. People who suffer from this disease are intolerant of gluten. They need gluten-free diet products. People who do not always have celiac disease may experience certain ailments from an early age, and for some, impaired nutrient uptake has been associated since infancy.

Oats, millet, buckwheat, brown rice, quinoa, chia seeds. All of these grains can be treated as gluten-free, as the gluten and other proteins (present in the grain) in these grains do not cause such an immune response in people with celiac disease as does the gluten in wheat, barley, and rye.

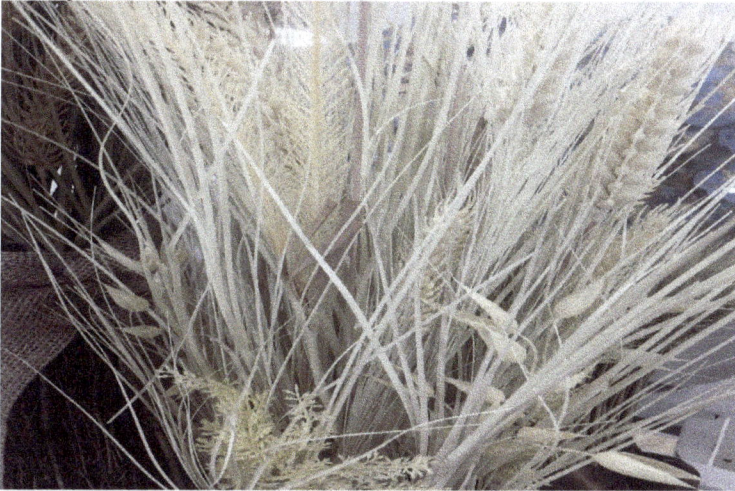

The main sources of carbohydrates are bread and its products. So, what to do for those who have to give up delicious bread and where to get the much-needed carbohydrates for the human body? As we have just found out, oatmeal, sorghum, millet, buckwheat, brown rice, and quinoa do not have dangerous gluten. Therefore, if you want to bake bread at home or make homemade pasta, you can boldly make flour mixtures from these grains by mixing them together at your own discretion. You can also boldly taste fruits, vegetables, meat (pure, except for some meat products).

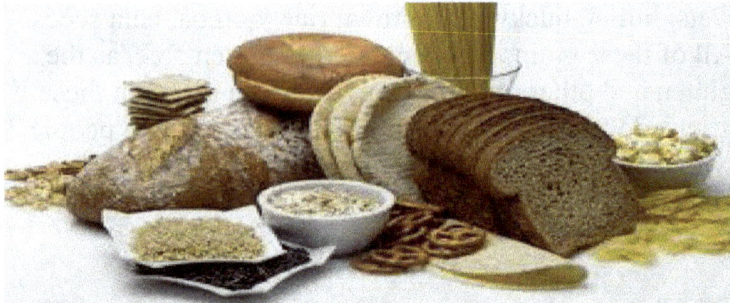

Most of the public has heard or read gluten somewhere, but don't know what it is. According to one survey, when people were asked what gluten was, the most common answer was "Gluten is a bad thing and should be avoided." The basic rule everyone should know is that gluten is a protein found in grains such as wheat, barley, and rye. When gluten enters the body, it can cause symptoms such as abdominal pain, bloating, rash, fatigue, and other gastrointestinal problems. The goal for people with celiac disease, gluten intolerance, or sensitivity is to completely get rid of gluten in their diet.

**Advertising Trick**

Starting a gluten-free diet may not result in weight loss. Gluten-free products are already very popular. Sometimes such products contain much higher levels of carbohydrates than usual. One example is a packet of gluten-free cookies that contain 60 calories in each cookie, which is more than a regular sandwich. Some products are made from gluten-free grains that are cleaned. Food fibers and other useful nutrients are usually removed from cleaned grains, making them less nutritious.

## The Relationship Between Quantity and Quality

To keep a nutritious diet, food needs to be balanced in a comprehensive way, especially in terms of quantity and quality.

If you consume gluten-free foods like, say brown rice, but consume them in large quantities, your weight will still grow. Simply put, your body is unable to process an excessive amount of food and so stores it.

If you have celiac disease or intolerance to gluten, you should choose each product and meal carefully, as gluten can "hide" everywhere. A few examples: it can be in your cosmetics- especially in lipstick, it can be in your salad dressing or in food supplements. Even some toothpastes have gluten.

Eat only as much food as your body can process and eat foods that do not even contain traces of gluten if you have intolerance.

Distinguish between the two terms "gluten-free and "wheat-free"

A bread labeled wheat-free does not mean it is gluten-free. The bread may contain other grains that have gluten.

If you do not have celiac disease and are not sensitive to gluten, removing gluten from your diet still will improve your well-being and beautify your body lines.

Consuming coarse grains will create a feeling of satiety, provide more energy, and help regulate your blood sugar and insulin. Consequently, your well-being will improve by removing gluten from your diet and changing some eating habits.

**Cooking With Grains**

Traditional dishes made from buckwheat grain or flour were considered as commoner food, however, many of these dishes are biologically valuable and they are very much loved now.

Porridge is prepared from grain, and so too are baked pudding, flat cakes, pies, and pancakes. Before preparing the dishes, the grains are washed, and the small grains are sifted again.

Grain porridges should be boiled. Some prefer to cook them until they are completely dry, though others prefer leaving thinner with more liquid content.

**Dry** grains are generally cooked with water, while water diluted with milk or broth is also typical.

**Thick** porridges are boiled in water diluted with milk, and less often in water. Porridge is stirred constantly so that it will not burn. Take 1 glass of grains, 2-4 glasses of water (take 2 glasses for buckwheat grains, 3 glasses for rice, and 4 glasses for pellets).

**Thin** grain porridges are cooked in milk (or in milk with water). Take 1 glass of grain and 4-5 glasses of milk (or milk diluted with water).

Porridge perfectly suits a full-fledged breakfast and reduces the tendency of overeating. By eating porridges and other meals from grains we get a minimum of 15 essential ingredients for the body: vitamins, minerals, carbohydrates, and vegetable fats. Research has shown that people who eat porridge in the morning eat healthier, less caloric snacks, and find it easier to maintain a healthy weight.

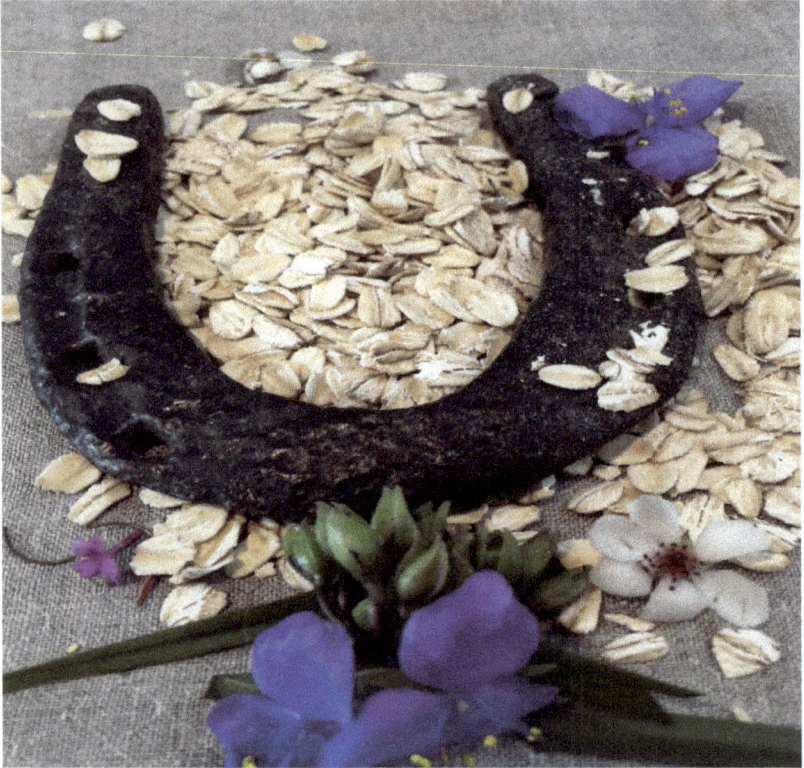

**Oats**

*"A grain, which in England is generally given to horses, but in Scotland supports the people."*
- Samuel Johnson  18th century writer, editor, and lexicographer.

Oats (Avena sativa). Oats are usually eaten in the form of oatmeal porridge or as baked wares such as oat biscuits. Oat porridge has a well-earned reputation for its health benefits. 100 g of oats contains 66.3 g of carbohydrates, which will give you enough energy to start your day. Oats provide a natural source of dietary fiber, which can help reduce the amount of bad cholesterol in our bodies. Oats contain a significant amount of B vitamins and are also a great source of minerals.

**Oats and allergy.** If you notice a dripping nose after eating an oatmeal porridge this is not necessarily a coincidence. If similar symptoms recur on a regular basis, it may be an allergy, or intolerance to the specific protein in oats. It is called avenin.

**Health Benefits of Oats**

Oats can reduce the risk of cardiovascular diseases. A Harvard study found that people who ate a bowl of oatmeal on a daily basis had a 20% lower risk of heart failure. The fibers in oats reduce cholesterol levels. Rich in beta glucan, oats protect the immune system against bacteria and microbes. Oats reduce the risk of cancer, reduce blood pressure, regulate blood sugar, and help with gastrointestinal disorders.

## Oatmeal Porridge with Berries

**Ingredients:** 750 ml (3 cups) of water, 1 cup of oatmeal, 2 teaspoons of butter, a pinch of salt, 200 g (5-6 tablespoons) of fresh or frozen berries.

**Preparation:** Boil water, add oat flakes to the water, salt, brew, and stir the porridge until it thickens. Remove from the heat, add some berries and stir the porridge. Pour into small bowls and decorate with the rest of the berries.

You can add a small piece of butter on top of the porridge. Pouring sweet milk over your bowl of porridge oats can also liven up the recipe.

## Oatmeal Cookies

**Ingredients:** 2 cups oatmeal, 2 cups all-purpose flour, 1 teaspoon baking soda, (1 cup) unsalted butter at room temperature, 1 cup brown sugar, or less (to taste), 2 eggs, 1 teaspoon vanilla extract, Optional: ½ teaspoon cinnamon, ½ cloves, ½ nutmeg, 2 tablespoons dried cranberries.

**Preparation:** Chop oats in food processor until fine, add flour, and 1 teaspoon baking soda, mix together. To room temperature butter, add brown sugar and mix together until fluffy, add eggs and vanilla extract into the butter mixture, swirl until incorporated. Blend in flour mixture and cranberries. Spread butter on the baking tray to keep cookies from sticking. Scoop the cookie dough out with a small ice-cream scoop, or by tablespoon, take in hands and roll into a ball. Place the cookie balls side by side on a baking tray and bake in a preheated oven at

350 degrees F (180 C) for 15-20 minutes until the oatmeal cookies become light brown. For extra decoration, consider adding chocolate drops or sprinkled coconut flakes. The oatmeal cookie dough can contain other ingredients, such as dried berries, fruits, nuts or sunflower or pumpkin seeds. seeds (e.g., sunflower or pumpkin seeds.

## Oatmeal Hamburgers

**Ingredients:** 400 g oatmeal, 1 egg, 1 onion, and a pinch each of salt and pepper.
**Preparation:** Soak the oatmeal with hot water, cover, and leave to swell for five minutes. Drain and put into a mixing bowl. Add an egg, chopped onion, pepper, and salt. Mix everything well and place with the spoon in a heated pan with oil. Bake until both sides of the hamburgers are browned. Hamburgers can be served as a main dish hot with white sauce, boiled potatoes, and salad, or cold.

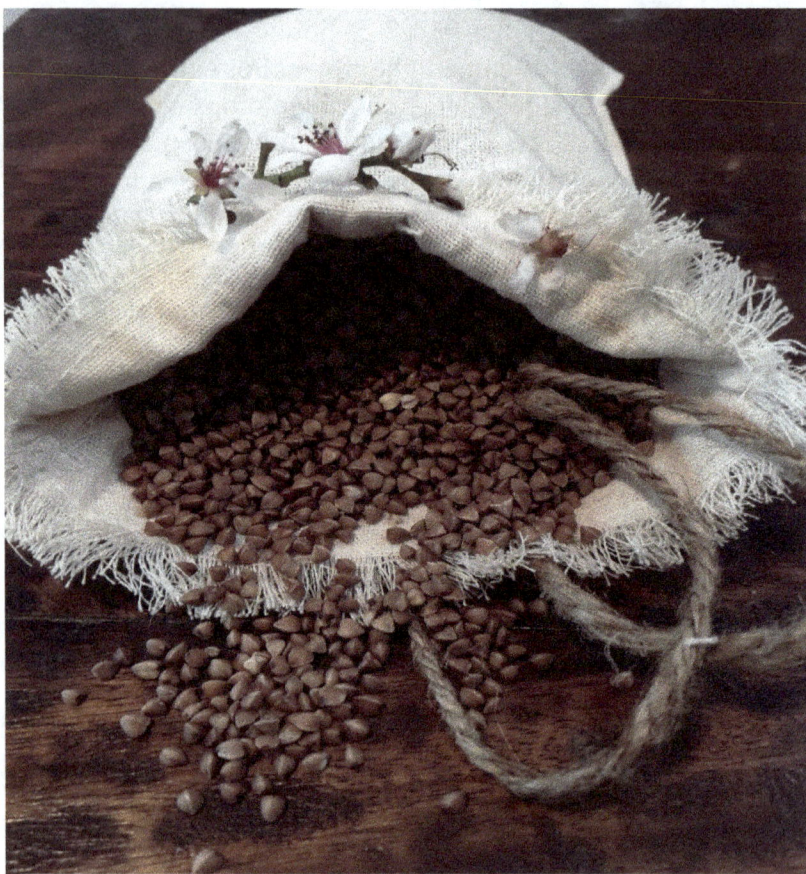

**Buckwheat**

"We're not wheat, we're buckwheat! When a storm comes along it flattens ripe wheat because it's dry and can't bend with the wind. But ripe buckwheat's got sap in it and it bends. And when the wind has passed, it springs up almost as straight and strong as before."
Margaret Mitchell – Author of "Gone with the Wind"

Buckwheat (Fagopyrum esculentum). The first
buckwheat crops are thought to have been grown 8,000
years ago in Southern China and the Himalayas when
buckwheat was the main source of food for the local
people. Later, buckwheat was replaced by rice and other
grain crops. Buckwheat has many names. In India, it is
called black rice; in France, Spain, and Belgium it is
called Arabian grain, and in Greece and Italy, buckwheat
is called Turkish grain.

**Health Benefits of Buckwheat**

Buckwheat is a source of vitamin B, nutrients, and
minerals. There are 343 calories in 100 g of buckwheat.
Buckwheat is a great source of energy. A good way to
start your day is with buckwheat porridge. Though not a
true cereal but a fruit, buckwheat seeds resemble cereal
grains and are often used just as one would use rice,
barley, bulgur, or quinoa, usually as a side dish.

The high potassium and iron present in buckwheat
prevent the body from absorbing radioactive isotopes
and the formation of blood clots, in addition to reducing
cholesterol. The mineral magnesium relaxes the blood
vessels, improves circulation, facilitates the transfer of
nutrients and lowers blood pressure. Buckwheat contains
a large amount of folic acid, which stimulates blood flow
and strengthens the body's resistance to adverse
environmental influences.

Buckwheat has many health-enhancing properties, with cardiovascular-improving properties prominent. Nutrients such as dietary fiber, potassium, and rutin contribute the most to this. Studies in China have shown that consuming at least 100 grams of buckwheat a day lowers total cholesterol, lowers low-density lipoprotein (LDL) cholesterol, which has been linked to cardiovascular disease, and increases good (high-density lipoprotein - HDL) cholesterol, which is associated with better health. The mineral magnesium relaxes the blood vessels, improves blood circulation, facilitates the transfer of nutrients and lowers blood pressure. Buckwheat has more protein than rice, wheat, millet, and quinoa.

**Energy source** - Research has been conducted in China on buckwheat, oats, wheat and sweet potatoes as energy sources. Buckwheat, along with oatmeal and wheat, are better sources of energy than sweet potatoes. 100 grams of buckwheat contains 343 calories.

**Blood Glucose** - Another study in China looked at the effects of buckwheat protein on blood glucose in the presence of a toxic glucose analog called alloxan. Alloxan destroys insulin-producing cells in the pancreas and causes symptoms similar to type 1 diabetes. Studies have shown that buckwheat protein was effective in lowering blood glucose. Buckwheat's high fiber content helps lower blood glucose.

**Blood pressure** - Animal studies conducted in Korea to test the effects of fresh and sprouted buckwheat on blood pressure showed that sprouted buckwheat reduced blood pressure more than fresh. However, using both fresh and sprouted buckwheat, less oxidative damage to aortic cells was observed.

**Cholesterol** - Buckwheat is one of the best sources of dietary fiber, which is an effective natural means of lowering blood cholesterol.

**Digestion** - Dietary fiber is one of the most important nutrients to support the good functioning of the digestive system. They help food move more easily through the intestines, keep the intestines clean and help prevent constipation. Dietary fiber is also associated with a lower risk of colon and rectal cancer.

**Buckwheat can cause allergic reactions in some people**, such as skin reactions, respiratory symptoms, and gastrointestinal symptoms.

**To prepare buckwheat**, mix 1 glass of grain and 2½ glasses of water or broth the evening before and soak overnight. Drain, then pour the mixture into salted boiling water. Reduce heat, stirring until the grains are swollen, then cover and simmer for two to three minutes.

**Buckwheat Salad with Zucchini, Carrots and Feta Cheese**

**Ingredients:** 100 g (4 ounces) of buckwheat, 4 glasses of water, 1 medium-sized carrot, 1 zucchini, 1 clove of garlic, a pinch of ground cumin, cilantro, turmeric, salt, black pepper, feta cheese, butter or oil.

**Preparation:** Rinse buckwheat with water two or three times and drain well. Soak the grains overnight in 4 glasses of water. In the morning, pour off the water. In a frying pan, place butter or oil, add grated carrot, and zucchini, and stir fry for 8 minutes. Add the buckwheat and spices and cook for another 2-3 minutes. Transfer to a medium bowl, add feta cheese, and stir well.

## Buckwheat Porridge

**Ingredients:** 1.5 cups of buckwheat, 2 glasses of milk, 2 tablespoons of butter or olive oil, salt. Porridge fruits and nuts are excellent accompanies to porridge.

**Preparation:** Rinse buckwheat with water two or three times and drain well. Soak the grains overnight in 4 glasses of water. In the morning, pour off the water. Add 2 glasses of milk, butter, and salt to a saucepan to boil. Add the buckwheat and boil over medium heat, stirring occasionally until mixture begins to thicken and the buckwheat has absorbed all liquid. Cover, and allow to stand for 2-3 minutes.

## Cabbage Rolls with Buckwheat

**Ingredients:** 1 head white cabbage, 4 large potatoes, peeled, and finely grated, 1 onion chopped, 2 cloves garlic, 2 tablespoon butter, 1½ cup sour cream, 1 cup buckwheat rinsed two or three times with boiling water, and drained well.

**Preparation:** preheat oven 350F. Remove the core from cabbage. Place whole cabbage in a large pot filled with boiling salted water. Cover and cook for 3 minutes or until softened enough to pull off individual leaves. You will need about 18 leaves.

When leaves are cool enough to handle, use a paring knife to cut away the thick center stem from each leaf, without cutting all the way through. Chop the remaining cabbage and place it in the bottom of a casserole dish or Dutch oven.

Drain the potatoes in a sieve or cheesecloth, twisting until potatoes are dry. Transfer to a large bowl and mix with a little vitamin C powder (ascorbic acid), or lemon juice so they do not turn dark, and set aside.

Sauté the chopped onions in butter in a small skillet and fry them until tender. Add to the potatoes, mixing well.

Add ½ cup sour cream, chopped garlic, and rinsed and drained buckwheat to potato mixture, combining thoroughly. Season to taste with salt and pepper.

Place about ½ cup of filling on each cabbage leaf. Roll away from you to encase the filling. Flip the right side of the leaf to the middle, then flip the left side. You will have something that looks like an envelope. Once again, roll away from you to create a neat little roll.

Place the cabbage roll on top of the chopped cabbage in the casserole dish or Dutch oven, seasoning each layer with pepper.

Pour 1 cup sour cream over the cabbage rolls, cover, and place in the oven. Bake for 1 to 1½ hours, or until buckwheat filling is tender.

Serve with pan juices or hot tomato sauce and more sour cream if desired, or mix the pan juice with sour cream, ladle it over the cabbage rolls.

**Tips**. They can be eaten hot or at room temperature. Mini cabbage rolls make great appetizers. Just spear them with a frilled toothpick and you are good to go. Cabbage rolls freeze well, before or after cooking, and can be made in a slow cooker (Look for manufacturing instructions).

## Buckwheat with Shrimp.

**Ingredients:** 1 cup buckwheat groats, pinch black pepper, bay leaves to taste, 1 red diced paprika, 1 carrot, 200 gm or 7 oz shrimp without shells (about 5 big or 6-10 small), salt, 8 oz vegetable broth, 200 gm (one bunch) asparagus, 6 oz or 170 gm of mushrooms, 1 tablespoon sunflower oil.

**Preparation**: In a casserole pot add asparagus, diced pepper, uncooked shrimp, sliced carrot, 1 tablespoon sunflower oil, vegetable broth, bay leaves, pepper, and salt. Bake at 350 F for 40 minutes.

## Buckwheat with Walnuts

**Ingredients:** ½ cup walnuts, 2 bananas, 2 stalks celery, 1 cup buckwheat groats, 4 teaspoons chia seeds.

**Preparation:** wash buckwheat groats two or three times with boiling water, drain well, add ⅕ cup of water and soak groats overnight. Next morning, drain the water and in a small pot boil the buckwheat for 2-3 minutes, drain well. In an electrical food processor add walnuts, bananas, celery, soaked chia seeds and grind for 5 minutes. Place in a small bowl and season with favorite fruits or berries.

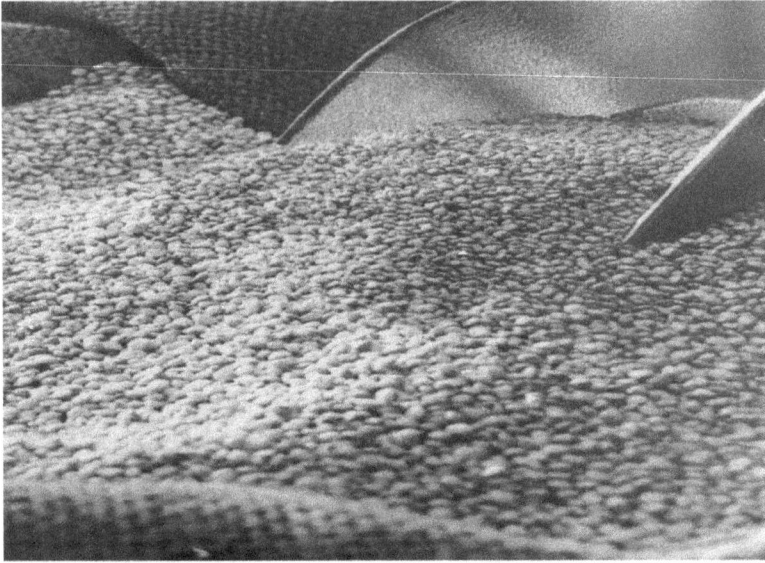

## Quinoa

*"Never eat ingredients you can't pronounce. Except quinoa. You should eat quinoa."*
- Yotam Ottolenghi – Israeli-born British chef

Quinoa (Chenopodium quinoa). This tiny nutty-tasting grain (pronounced "keen-wah") is an herbaceous annual plant grown as a grain crop primarily for its edible seeds. Quinoa originated in the Andean region of northwestern South America and was domesticated 3000 to 4000 years ago for human consumption in the Lake Titicaca basin of Peru and Bolivia, although archaeological evidence shows livestock use 7000 years ago. Quinoa provides protein, dietary fiber, B vitamins, and dietary minerals in rich amounts above those of wheat, corn, rice or oats. It is gluten-free. Quinoa is also used in cosmetics.

Quinoa can be eaten as a hot porridge with spice or sweet porridge with milk (coconut, soy, almond), yogurt, honey, nuts, or fruits, or with greens as a salad. Quinoa is an excellent addition to soups and stews. Like rice, it goes well with meat and fish. Some types of noodles and flour are also made from quinoa. It is good for stuffings.

This plant does not belong to the cereal family, but its fruits are considered grains.

**Health Benefits of Quinoa**

Quinoa provides protein, dietary fiber, minerals, vitamins B, and vitamin E, low sugars, and saturated fat. In addition, the calcium and iron content are much higher in quinoa than in rice, corn, wheat, or oats. To increase the nutritional value of quinoa, it is best to sprout it for about 2-4 hours. Quinoa does not contain gluten. The nutritional value of quinoa per 100 gm is 356 kcal.

Quinoa is easy to prepare. First, rinse the seeds thoroughly in running cold water and then pour them into clean, cold, salted water. Mix 1 part of the grains with 2 parts of water or broth and bring to boil on a medium heat. Reduce to a simmer for 10-15 minutes or until tender and the liquid absorbed. The boiled quinoa increases significantly in volume and changes its shape as the grains become crispy.

Quinoa can substitute for oats in recipes. Boiled grains mixed with fruits, nuts, or honey form an excellent breakfast. Quinoa is often used in vegetarian dishes for its texture.

**Some people have cause allergic reaction to quinoa,** such as stomach aches, itching skin, hives or other common symptoms of food allergies.

### Quinoa and Parsley Salad

**Ingredients:** 1½ cup of water, ¾ cup of quinoa, ½ cup or less of lemon juice, 1 tablespoon of olive oil, ⅓ glass of thinly sliced parsley leaves, one small cucumber, salt, and pepper.
**Preparation:** Wash the quinoa well and boil. If there is still water left in the grains after boiling, filter it, add salt and pepper (according to taste), sliced cucumber, and parsley and mix. To garnish the dish, add a dash of lemon juice with olive oil over the top.

### Cherry Walnut Quinoa Salad

**Ingredients:** 2 glasses of milk, 8 oz of quinoa, 12 oz of halved and pitted (can also be frozen) cherries, ½ glass of walnuts, 4 tablespoons of liquid honey, ½ teaspoons of cinnamon, 3 tablespoons plain yogurt, 1½ tbsp of chia seeds.
**Preparation:** Rinse the quinoa with water and boil with 2 glasses of milk. Reduce the heat and simmer for about 15 minutes or until tender. Put walnuts, cherries, and

cinnamon with the boiled quinoa, let it cool a little bit, pour yogurt, add honey. Mix thoroughly, and top with sprinkled chia seeds.

People who are allergic to honey, fruits, or other ingredients found in these grain dishes should **not eat** the salad.

**Tabbouleh -** The wonderful classic refreshing Middle Easter salad.

**Ingredients:** 1½ cups quinoa, 2.5 cups water, 1 large bunch of spring onions thinly sliced, 1 cucumber finely chopped or diced, 3 tomatoes chopped, 1.5-2.5 ml / ¼ - ½ tsp ground cumin, 1 large bunch chopped fresh flat leaf parsley, 1 large bunch chopped fresh mint, juice of 2 lemons, or to taste, 60 ml / 4 tbsp extra virgin olive oil, romaine lettuce leaves, olives, lemon wedges, tomato wedges, cucumber slices, and mint springs to garnish (optional). Natural (plain) yogurt to serve (optional).
**Preparation:** Rinse the quinoa well with cold water, drain, and place it to boil with 2.5 cups water. Boil in a medium heat saucepan over high heat. Reduce heat to medium-low, cover, and simmer until quinoa is tender. Remove from the heat, and let stand, covered, for 5 minutes. If there is still water left in the grains after boiling, filter it. Fluff with a fork. Add the spring onions to the quinoa wheat, then mix and squeeze together with your hands to combine. Add the cucumber, tomatoes, cumin, parsley, mint, lemon and oil to the quinoa wheat and toss well. Heap the tabbouleh onto a bed of lettuce

leaves and garnish with olives, lemon wedges, tomato, cucumber and mint sprigs. Serve with a bowl of natural yogurt.

**Quinoa, Fresh Figs, and Honey-Parfait**.

**Ingredients:** 1 cup water, ½ cup quinoa, 1 tsp vanilla extract, ¼ ground Ceylon cinnamon, 8 fresh figs, 1 cup vanilla yogurt ¼ cup honey, chia seeds, ½ tsp lemon juice.
**Preparation:** In a small saucepan, bring water to a boil. Add quinoa, reduce heat, simmer, covered until liquid is absorbed, 15-20 minutes. Remove from heat, let it cool. Layer half of quinoa mixture, half of honey, half of figs, and half of yogurt into 4 parfait glasses. Top with remaining quinoa mixture, honey, chia seeds, and figs. Sprinkle with lemon juice.

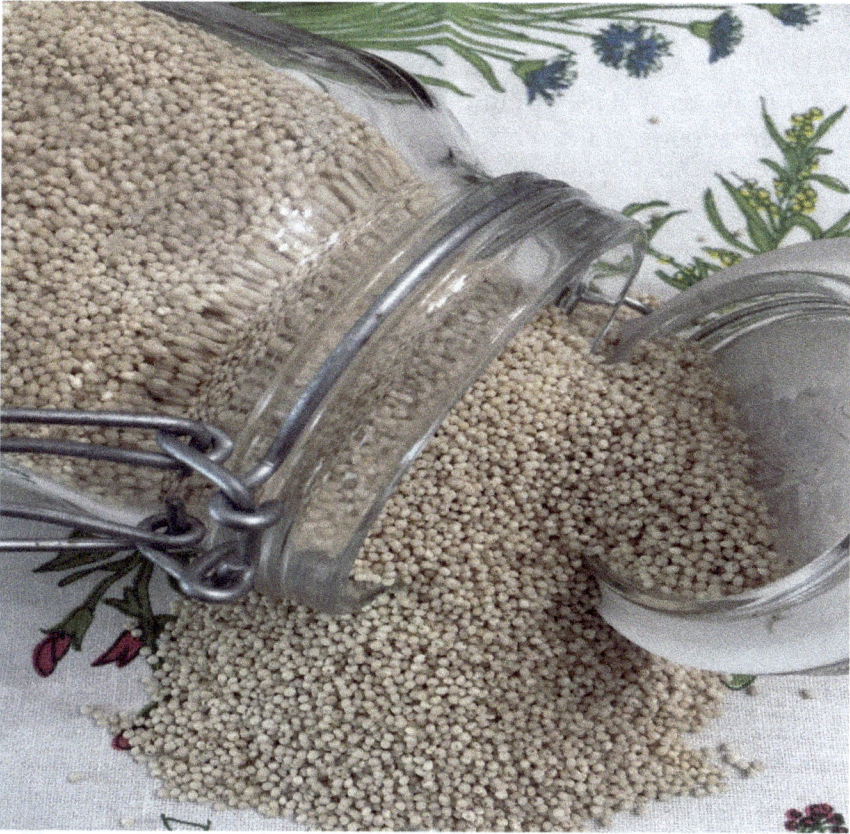

**Millet**

*Good millet is known at the harvest.*
- Proverb from Kenya

Little millet domesticated in India (Panicium sumatrence) is a gluten free grain alternative to wheat.

The origin of millet (also called ragi) is debated with various proposals placing it in Abyssinia, Africa, or India. Various species of millet have been domesticated in different parts of the world, most notably in Asia and Africa. In Ethiopia, millet has been consumed since prehistoric times. Millets also formed important parts of the prehistoric diet in India. The Indian flatbread roti is made from ground millet seeds. In the Middle Ages, before potatoes and corn were introduced, millet became a staple in Europe, especially in Eastern Europe. Millet was introduced into the United States in the 19th century. Millet is a starchy, protein rich grain. One cup of cooked millet has 207 calories and is rich with copper, phosphorus, manganese, and magnesium. Organic millet is the only alkaline grain and contains all the essential amino acids. It is a rich source of silicon, which helps build collagen for healthy skin, eyes, nails, and arteries.

The majority of the world's commercial millet crop is produced by India, China, Nigeria, Greece, and Egypt.

**Health Benefits of Millet**

Millet is starchy, protein rich grain. One cup of cooked millet has 207 calories. Rich with copper, phosphorus, manganese, magnesium, vitamins, packed with protein, antioxidants and nutrients, it even reduces blood sugar and cholesterol levels. It is especially helpful in keeping type 2 diabetes under control, protecting the immune system, and can reduce the risk of cardiovascular diseases, while calming gastrointestinal disorders.

Cooked millet can be served as a breakfast porridge. Try adding some of your favorite fruits or nuts. For a lunch or dinner meal, make a salad and top it with fried eggs.

**Garlic, Spinach, and Eggs**

**Ingredients:** ½ cup millet, ¼ teaspoon sea salt, ¼ teaspoon black pepper, ½ teaspoon unsalted butter, 1 clove minced garlic, 2-3 handfuls of shredded spinach, 2 large eggs, 3-4 tablespoons hummus, and to top: olive oil and black pepper.

**Preparation:** like all grains, before cooking millet rinse it thoroughly under running water and remove any debris you may find. After rinsing, add one part millet to two a half parts boiling water or broth. After the liquid has returned to a boil, turn down the heat, cover and simmer for about 25 minutes. This way the texture of millet will be fluffy like rice. If you want the millet to have a creamier consistency, stir it frequently with a little water.

In a dry saucepan, cook millet over medium-low heat for 3-4 minutes. Pour 1 cup of water into the pot, bring to boil, reduce to low, cover, and let simmer until the majority of water is absorbed, roughly 15 minutes. Remove from heat, still covered, and let sit while preparing remaining parts of the meal. Heat butter in a skillet over low heat and add minced garlic. Cook for 1-2 minutes until the garlic is fragrant. Add spinach and turn off the heat. Stir and let sit until spinach is mostly wilted. Stir in millet and transfer to plates. In the same skillet, fry eggs and place on top of the millet. Top with a dollop of hummus, drizzle of olive oil, and sprinkle of bleach pepper.

**Moroccan Carrot Salad with Millet.** This Moroccan spice blend (Ras El Hanout) is easily made with spices you most likely have on hand.

**Ingredients:** ½ pound carrots sliced round, ½ cup sliced red onion, 1 tablespoon olive oil, 2 teaspoons Moroccan spice blend (Ras El Hanout), ½ cup uncooked millet, ¼ cup sliced almonds, ¼ cup pomegranate seeds, ¼ cup flat leaf minced parsley, 2 tablespoons minced cilantro, one lemon juice, 2 tablespoon olive oil, Kalamata olives. If you do not have carrots, sweet potatoes would be a good option followed closely by parsnip (for flavor).
**Preparation**: Preheat the oven to 375F. Cut in round slices of carrots. Place on a baking sheet covered with parchment paper and toss with onions, 1 tablespoon olive oil, and spice bland. Roast carrots until brown and tender, 20-25 minutes. While the carrots are roasting, combine millet with 1 cup water and a pinch of salt. Bring to a boil, reduce to simmer, cover, and cook for 18 minutes or until most of the water has been absorbed.

Remove from heat and allow it to sit for 5 minutes. In a bowl, combine the roasted carrots, millet, almond slices, pomegranate seeds, and herbs. Squeeze lemon juice over salad followed by 2 tablespoons olive oil, adding more as desired. Toss together, taste, and add salt and pepper to taste.

You could toss the final mixture with lettuce or fresh spinach. Before you toss greens let the millet cool. To further ramp up the protein provided by this dish, try adding chickpeas or feta cheese.

## Chickpea Shawarma with Millet

**Ingredients:** 2 cups raw chickpeas or 1.5 oz can, drained and rinsed, 3 cloves minced garlic, 1 tablespoon ground cumin, 1 tablespoon ground coriander, 1 teaspoon sea salt, 1 teaspoon turmeric powder, 1 teaspoon allspice, ½ teaspoon ground ginger, ½ teaspoon black pepper, pinch of cayenne pepper, 3 tablespoons olive oil, ⅓ cup thinly sliced red onion, 1 cup uncooked millet, 2 cups water, pinch of salt.

Toppings: flat leaves of parsley, roasted red pepper, hummus, feta cheese, diced red onions.

**Preparation:** Preheat the oven to 350F. In a medium bowl, combine minced garlic with spices (cumin, cayenne pepper). Add in the olive oil and stir until well combined. Stir in the chickpeas and red onion. Transfer to a roasted pan and cover with foil. Bake for 30 minutes until onions are tender. When chickpeas are finished cooking, place in a pot with 2 cups of water and a pinch of salt. Bring to boil, reduce to a simmer, and let cook until the majority of water has been absorbed (12-15 minutes). Cover, remove from heat, and let sit until chickpeas are tender. Divide the millet into servings, cover with chickpeas, and add your favorite toppings, such as tomatoes, cucumbers, or yogurt sauce.

## Millet Cake with Carrots and Spinach

**Ingredients:** 1 cup millet, rinsed, 2 cups water, pinch of salt and pepper, 3 teaspoons olive oil, 1 shallot, minced, 6 ounces (6 cups) baby spinach, chopped, 2 carrots, peeled and shredded, 2 garlic cloves, minced, 2 teaspoons curry powder, ¼ cup plain yogurt, 1 tablespoon almond milk, 1 large egg, lightly beaten, ¼ cup ground flaxseed, 2 tablespoons minced cilantro, any sauce or chutney you like - I topped mine with Greek yogurt, mixed with salt, pepper, chile flakes, and a squeeze of lime or lemon.

**Preparation:** preheat the oven to 350 F and line a large baking sheet with parchment paper. Combine the millet, water, and ½ teaspoon salt in a medium saucepan and bring to simmer over medium heat. Reduce heat to low, cover and simmer until grains are tender and liquid is absorbed, about 15-20 minutes. Turn off the heat, let millet sit, covered, for 10 minutes, transfer to a large bowl. Heat 1 tablespoon olive oil in a ½ inch nonstick skillet over medium heat until shimmering. Add the shallot and cook until softened, about 3 minutes. Stir in the spinach and carrots and cook until spinach wilts, about 2 minutes. Stir in the garlic, curry powder, ½ teaspoon salt, ¼ teaspoon pepper and cook until fragrant, about 30 seconds. Transfer the mixture to the bowl with millet. Add the yogurt, egg (or flax plus almond milk), and cilantro into the millet mixture and fold until well combined. Use a ⅓ cup measuring cup to scoop the mixture, then form into a half-inch thick cake, and place in the prepared sheet. Repeat. Refrigerate cake until chilled and firm, about 30 minutes (15 minutes for the vegan version). Drizzle the cake with olive and bake for

20-30 minutes or until the edges are crispy and the cake is cooked through.
This can be served for breakfast or a meal. Simply delicious, healthy, and refreshing.

**Millet Dals**

**Ingredients:** ½ cup millet, 1 ½ cups water, salt as needed, 1 ½ tablespoon sunflower oil(use as needed), ½ tablespoon mustard seeds, ⅓ cup bengal gram (chana dal) - chickpea lentils, ⅔ cup skinned black gram (urad dal) - black lentil, ¼ cup peanuts or cashews split (use as needed), pinch asafetida ( hing) - as a spice powder (you could buy in a grocery shops), 1 green chili, split, 1 red chili broken, ⅛ tsp turmeric, 1 tsp. Ginger grated, 1 sprig curry leaves, 1 lemon medium to large (use as needed). (Note: Hing or heeng is the Hindi word for asafetida (sometimes spelled asafoetida). It's also been known as the devil's dung and stinking gum, as well as asant, food of the gods, jowani badian, hengu, ingu, kayam, and ting. It is a dark brown, resin-like substance that is derived from the root of ferula. (Asafetida is used in savory dishes, often to add a more full flavor. It is a staple ingredient in Indian cooking. Commonly used along with turmeric in lentil dishes like dal and a variety of vegetable dishes)

**Preparation:** Add ½ cup millet into the pot and wash thoroughly. Drain completely. Add 1½ cups water to the pot and allow to soak for a while. Cook on a medium heat until all water is absorbed, but slightly soggy. Cover the pot and simmer on the lowest heat until completely cooked. Fluff gently with a fork and cool completely. Heat the pot with sunflower oil. Add mustard seeds, and when they begin to splutter, add chana dal (chickpea lentils), urad dal (black lentils), cashews, red chili, and green chili. When the dals turn slightly golden, add curry leaves, ginger, and green chili. Curry leaves turn crispy quickly. Then add turmeric, and pinch asafetida. Pour 3-4 tbsp water and cook until all of the water evaporates. This will bring out the aroma of the spices and soften the dals slightly. For even softer dals, use 1-2 tablespoon more water. Turn off the heat. Add the cooled millets and squeeze in lemon juice. Mix everything well. Serve lemon millet with curd or vegetable salad.

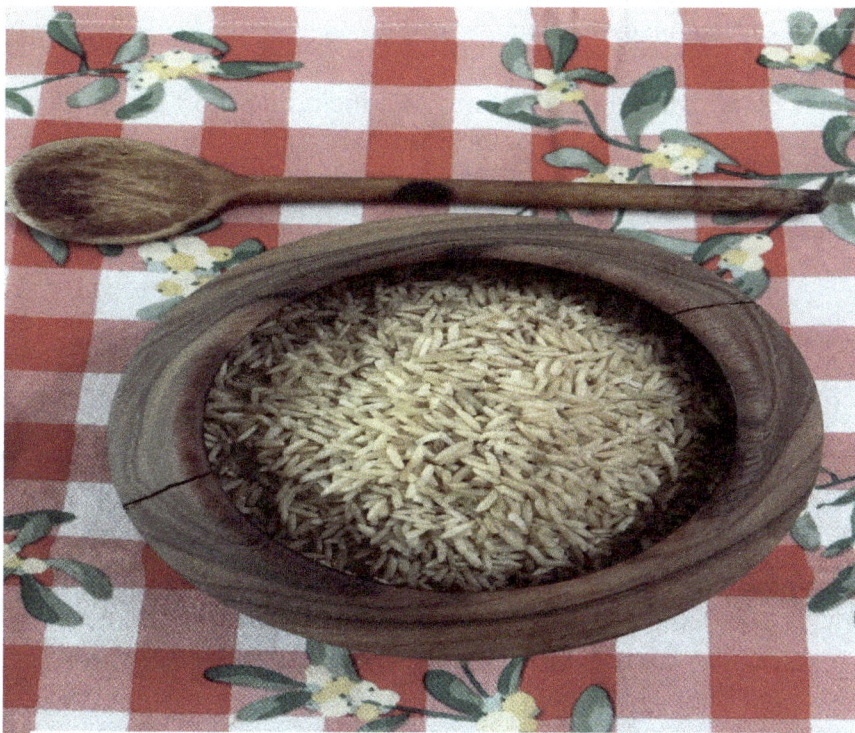

**Rice:**

*Rice is the best, the most nutritive, and unquestionably the most widespread staple in the world.*
- Auguste Escoffier – 19th century culinary artist

Rice (Ozyra sativa) commonly known as Asian rice. Rice occurs in a variety of colors, including white, brown, black, and red.

Rice comes in several varieties including short grain, medium grain, and long grain. Varieties include Indonesia black rice and Thai jasmine black rice. It has a nutty flavor, and the size of the grain gives each variety a unique texture once cooked. Brown rice also takes longer to cook compared to refined white rice. **Brown rice has a shelf life of approximately 6 months.**

Short grain Japonica variety grain (sometimes called sinica) is a sticky, brown rice, short, plump, and almost round in appearance. The grains are soft, tender, and stick together when cooked.

Medium grain brown rice is larger and plumper compared to short-grain, but not as large as the long-grain variety. The grains are very moist and tender, with less tendency to stick together when cooked compared to the short-grain variety.

Long grain brown rice is long and slender, and less sticky compared to the medium and short-grain varieties. Japanese variety long grained indica rice are usually cultivated in dry fields (except that in Japan it is cultivated mainly submerged). It is also the most familiar variety used in popular dishes like rice pilaf. The grains are light, fluffy, and separate easily when cooked.

## Health Benefits of Rice

Brown rice is a popular gluten-free, whole grain option for those diagnosed with celiac disease, wheat sensitivity, or non-celiac gluten sensitivity. It also contains valuable phytochemicals shown to play a valuable role in disease prevention.

Brown rice is nutritious. A great source of phosphorus, iron, zinc, rice is high in fiber, vitamins, minerals, antioxidants, rich in carbs and protein, and has minimal sugar. Many of the health benefits of brown rice come from the antioxidants, fiber, and other valuable chemical compounds.

Research has indicated that brown rice is associated with a wide range of helpful medicinal properties. Studies indicate brown rice as an important compound of a healthy diet and promotes a reduced risk of chronic diseases such as diabetes. It improves heart health, digestive health, reduces certain cancer risks, improves cholesterol levels, decreases inflammation, and can help with weight loss.

### A note about arsenic

Arsenic is a toxin occurring naturally in the environment. It is also found in nearly all foods and drinks to some degree, including brown rice. According to Consumer Reports, rice tends to absorb arsenic more readily than many other plants. Regular exposure to small amounts of arsenic can increase the risk of bladder, lung, and skin cancer, as well as heart disease and type 2 diabetes.

There are two different types of arsenic—organic and inorganic—the latter being the most toxic form. Higher levels of inorganic arsenic have been found in brown rice because of contaminated irrigation water. Sometimes cooking water is the cause of increased inorganic arsenic levels in brown rice.

**Suggestions to reduce the levels of arsenic in brown rice include:**
Wash brown rice in filtered water low in arsenic before cooking.
Cook brown rice in plenty of filtered water low in arsenic. (6 to 1 water to rice ratio is best)
If you eat large amounts of rice, white rice may be a better option than brown rice.
Vary the type of grains consumed during the week.
**Eat brown rice in moderation as part of a varied diet.**


**Greek Brown Rice Salad**

**Ingredients:** 2 ¼ cups water, 1 cup dry brown rice, ½ teaspoon freshly ground black pepper, ¼ cup fresh lemon juice, ¼ extra-virgin olive oil, ⅔ cup chopped fresh herbs (basil, dill, mint, and parsley), ⅔ thinly sliced scallion greens (green parts only), 1 cup crumbled feta cheese, 2 cloves minced garlic, one yellow onion chopped, 2 cups cherry tomatoes, ⅓ cup chopped walnuts, ½ cucumber chopped, pinch salt.

**Preparation:** wash brown rice well and soak it for about 15-20 minutes in plenty of cold water, enough to cover the rice by one centimeter. Do not skip washing or soaking the rice well, this is important to help get rid of excess starch which causes rice to be sticky. Soaking the rice here also shortens the cooking time. When you finish the soaking, drain the rice, and leave it covered and undisturbed in the pot for about 10 minutes before adding the herbs. This helps maintain the texture and integrity of the rice.

In a medium saucepan, bring water to a boil over high heat. Stir in rice, reduce the heat, cover and simmer until rice is tender and water has been absorbed, 35-40 minutes. Remove from the heat, allow rice to steam for 5 minutes with the lid on. Then, remove the lid and allow the rice to cool until it is close to room temperature. Stir in the salt, pepper, lemon juice, olive oil, herbs, garlic, onion, scallion greens, feta cheese, cherry tomatoes, chopped walnuts, chopped cucumber. Serve promptly, or refrigerate tightly covered until serving.

## Chicken Fried Rice with Asparagus

**Ingredients:** 2 tablespoon peanut oil (with peanut allergies, make this with a different soft oil, such as sesame or avocado). Avoid olive oil, which is too strongly flavored for this dish.) 1 pound chicken breast, chopped into bite sized pieces, ½ yellow onion, peeled and chopped, 1 carrot, chopped, 3 garlic cloves, minced, 1 tablespoon minced ginger, 2 cups asparagus (approximately a 1 pound bunch), ⅓ cup water, 2 cups cooked brown rice, chilled, 2 tablespoons low sodium soy sauce, ¾ cup frozen green peas.

**Preparation:** heat 1 tbsp of the oil on medium-high heat in a large skillet. Add chicken and cook until golden on all sides, about 5 to 8 minutes. Remove chicken from the skillet and set aside in a bowl. Wipe skillet clean. Add remaining tablespoon oil to the skillet and heat on medium-high. Add onion, carrot, garlic, and ginger. Saute 2-3 minutes until the onion is translucent. Stir in asparagus and ⅓ cup water, scraping up any browned bits at the bottom. Cook until asparagus is tender but still bright green and water has evaporated, about 5 minutes. Stir in rice and soy sauce and cook, stirring occasionally, until slightly crispy and warmed through, about 5 minutes total. Stir in peas and cook an additional minute to warm through.

To make this dish vegan, swap cubes of tofu for the chicken. You may want to marinate the tofu first or toss with a seasoning spice, like lemon or pepper. For gluten free fried rice, use tamari instead of soy sauce. Tamari is a soy sauce made from only soybeans rather than a blend of soy and wheat. If you are allergic to soy, look for coconut aminos, which have a similar umami flavor. (Umami means pleasant savory taste. Umami was finally isolated in Japan, which is why it has a Japanese savory delicious flavor.) You could use any combination of vegetables, such as zucchini, green beans, broccoli, or peppers.

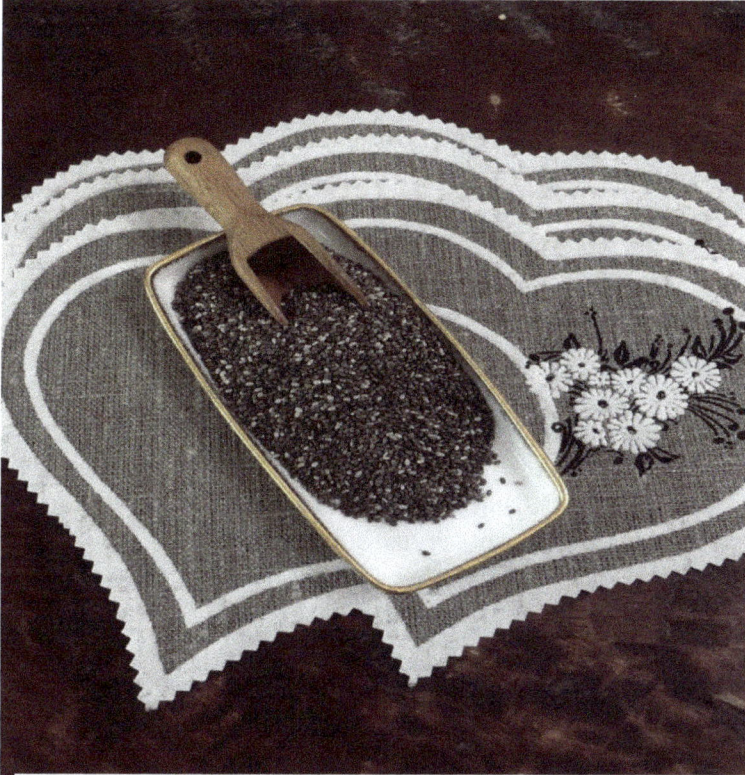

**Chia Seeds**

*Cooking with healthy and nutritious Chia seeds is just as much art as science. It is important to taste and investigate methods and foods in your own laboratory (your body) and observe how various things affect you.*
- Mantak Chia – 20th century Thai Taoist Master
-

Chia seeds (Salvia hispanica), in the mint family, are native to central and southern Mexico. There is evidence that the crop was widely cultivated by Aztecs in pre-Columbian times and was a staple food for Mesoamerican cultures. Ground or whole chia seeds are used for nutritional drinks and food. Chia seeds are cultivated and consumed in their ancestral homeland of Central Mexico, and commercially throughout Central and South America. It's also popular in Australia.

**Health Benefits of Chia Seeds**

Chia seeds are very rich in omega-3 fatty acids and are an excellent source of dietary fiber. Dried Chia seeds contain 6% water, 42% carbohydrates, 16% protein, and 31% fat. Chia seeds are a rich source of B vitamins, including thiamin, riboflavin, and folate. Dietary minerals they offer include calcium, iron, magnesium, manganese, phosphorus, and zinc.

Eating chia seeds can help cardiovascular risk factors, such as lowering cholesterol, and blood pressure. Its fiber stimulates digestion and increases energy levels. Being rich in protein helps boost mood. They're an excellent source of antioxidants, help in building strong bones, and promote oral health. They're delicious raw, non-GMO, and organic.

Chia seeds are used for nutrition drinks and food, mainly added to other foods as a topping or put into smoothies, breakfast cereals, energy bars, granola bars, yogurt, tortillas, overnight oats, soups, salads, and baked goods, like cakes and muffins, and even salad dressings for an extra boost of goodness. To get the most nutrients out of your food and to maximize the potential benefits of chia seed, soak them before adding them to a recipe or smoothie. They also may be made into gelatin.

Chia seeds can act as an egg substitute. For vegans and individuals with egg allergies, a chia egg can be a wonderful stand-in favorite baked good. When combined with liquid, the outer layer of the seed swells, and forms a gel. This makes chia seeds especially suited to replacing eggs in recipes for baked goods.

**Allergy**. Some people could have allergic reactions to chia, ranging from mild itching to more severe symptoms such as vomiting, diarrhea, or swelling of lips or tongue.

**Basic Chia Seed Preparation:** Add 1 tbsp chia seeds to a small dich and top with 2 ½ tbsp water. Stir, and let it rest for 5 minutes to thicken. It works well in pancakes, quick bread, muffins, cookies, and many other baked recipes.

**Chia Seeds Pudding.** This chia seeds pudding makes a very nice breakfast or dessert.

**Ingredients:** combine 6 tablespoons of chia seeds with 2 cups of nut milk, a teaspoon of vanilla, and 1 tablespoon of honey.

**Preparation**: allow to sit 1-2 hours in the refrigerator (or overnight), then divide into two servings, and enjoy with fresh fruit or some cacao nibs.

**Chia Seed Pudding with Strawberries**

**Ingredients:** 1 cup vanilla flavored almond milk, 1 cup plain low-fat 2% Greek yogurt, 6 tablespoon pure maple syrup, 1 teaspoon pure vanilla extract, ¼ cup chia seeds, 1 pint strawberries, hulled and chopped, and ¼ sliced almonds, toasted.

**Preparation:** In a medium bowl, gently whisk the almond milk with the yogurt. Add 2 tbsp maple syrup and 1 tsp vanilla and blend. Whisk in the chia seeds. Let stand for 30 minutes. Stir to distribute the seeds if they have settled. Cover and refrigerate overnight. The next day, in a medium bowl toss the berries with the remaining 4 teaspoons of maple syrup. Mix in the almonds. Spoon the pudding in 4 bowls or glasses, mount the berry mixture on top and serve.

**Smoothies and Shakes:** A couple of tablespoons can be added to shakes or smoothies to increase daily vitamins.

**Beverages.** Soak some chia seeds in lemon or lime juice to add some sparkle to summer iced tea.

## Seven Goodies from Nature.

*The greatest wealth is health*
-Virgil -1st century BC Latin philosopher

A balanced diet is an important part of a healthy lifestyle, and a few simple products can quickly and effectively strengthen the body's immune shield. Strong immunity helps prevent health ailments and makes it easier to overcome the diseases. When planning a big weekly shopping trip, a food production expert suggests paying attention to the seven immune-boosting benefits that nature offers to us. Focusing on these seven natural products and adding them more often to your menu and shopping lists will boost your natural immunity.

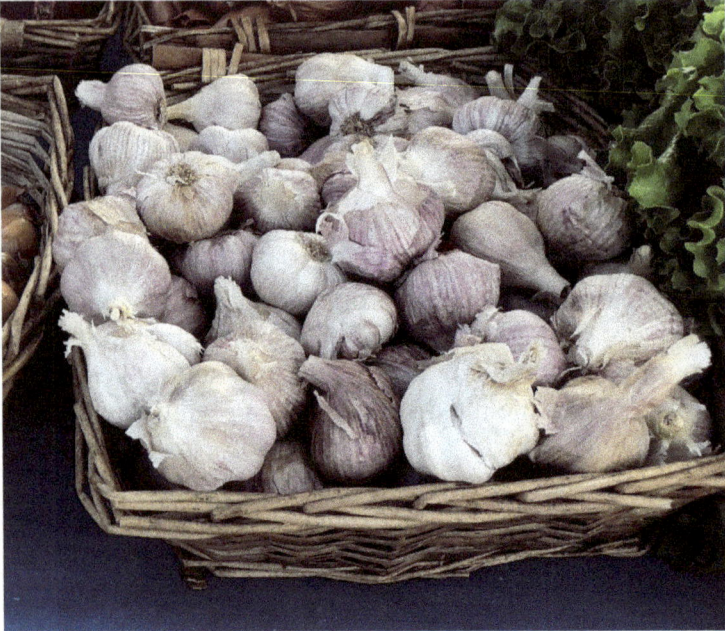

## Garlic

Garlic (Allium sativum) is a strong antibiotic. The ancient Egyptians, Greeks, and Romans all considered garlic a universal means of improving the body.

Garlic is a major ingredient in Indian cuisine. Garlic has been grown in Asia from immemorial times. The Italians, Greeks, Spanish, Jews, and French do not imagine food without garlic. It is said that a mixture of garlic, onions, and radishes was given to the builders of the pyramids. Garlic was a necessary entry to the gladiator's diet. Pythagoras called garlic "The king of spices" and the famous physician Avicenna knew thousands of recipes with garlic.

**Health Benefits of Garlic**

An active ingredient of garlic is called allicin. It is a powerful antibiotic that inhibits the ability for harmful bacteria from growing and multiplying in our bodies. Garlic slows the progression of cancer cells. Garlic reduces decay processes in the intestine, increases the functioning of gastric and small intestines, and promotes cardiovascular activity. The active substances of both garlic and lemon cleanse the body effectively. Garlic improves the skin's appearance, leaving it brighter, smoother, and more elastic. Garlic also is thought to cure acne and pigmentation spots and improves mood, reduces fatigue, strengthens immunity, and reduces blood pressure. Garlic is known as a remedy for intestinal parasites. Adding garlic to your curd of yogurt will help maintain the balance of good bacteria in the intestine. When a flu virus is spreading to your home or workplace, eat a few cloves of garlic with one tablespoon of apple jam (so as not to irritate the stomach). This will strengthen your immunity.

If you bought too much garlic, split it into slices, peel, and store them in a bowl of olive oil. Garlic will stay fresh for several months in the refrigerator, and the oil can be used for salad dressings.

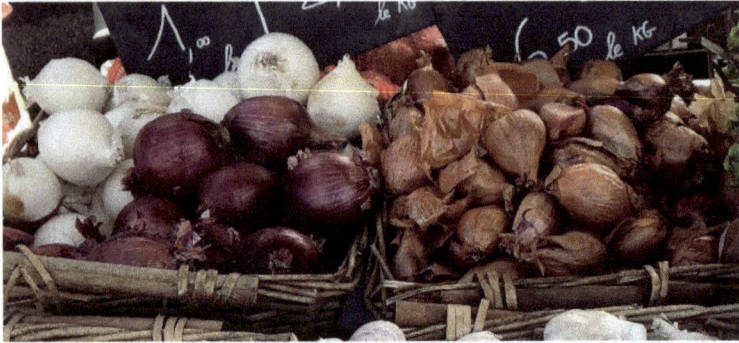

## Onions

Garden onion (Allium cepa). This plant spread very long ago in Egypt, Rome, and Greece. The homeland of the garden onion is Central Asia. The shepherds of Afghanistan, Iran, and Turkmenistan wandering through the mountain paths were the first to recognize that this plant was edible. The medicinal properties of onions were known in the ancient Eastern countries where the saying went, "Onion, when you touch me, any illness passes."

Onions have a sharp smell and taste due to irritating mucous quercetin glycosides. They contain plenty of enzymes, vitamins C, B1, B2, PP, carotenoids, saccharides, inulin, amino acids, pectins, microelements and other substances

Onion grows up to 60 cm high. Both lower and upper part of the onion is edible. The upper part of the onion, the greens, are called spring onions.

## Onion Healing Properties

Onions reduce blood pressure, cholesterol levels, stimulate blood circulation, protect against colds, and purify and strengthen the body.

1. Onion improves your overall body condition: eat 15-100 g of onion, stewed in steam, cooked in oven, or dried, twice a day, 15 minutes before eating your regular meals. Course duration: 2-3 weeks.

2. For impaired hearing or sight, drink fresh onion juice evenly mixed with honey, 1 teaspoonful 3-4 times a day, before each meal.

3. Treat insect stings with the grease from onion juice.

4. For hair loss and scalp scaling, scrub the scalp with fresh onion juice twice a week.

5. The active onion ingredients such as quercetin help to protect against cold and flu. Simply place a cut onion near the bed at night to prevent the accumulation of microbes through the air. When you have a stuffy nose, fold mashed onions into a few layers of gauze pieces, and hold it under your nose.

6. At the first signs of cold and flu: grease the mucous membrane with fresh onion juice or inhale their vapors 2-3 minutes for 3-4 times a day. If tolerated, place an onion juice saturated gauze directly into your nostrils for 10-15 minutes three times a day.

Onions are rich in substances that improve the absorption of calcium and magnesium, preventing infections by fungi and bacteria.

The best way to use the onion is fresh and uncooked, adding it to salads, sandwiches, soups, garnishes, sauces, and other dishes.

**Do not use onions** if you suffer from acute gastritis, duodenal ulcer, or inflammatory diseases of the intestinal, kidney, or liver.

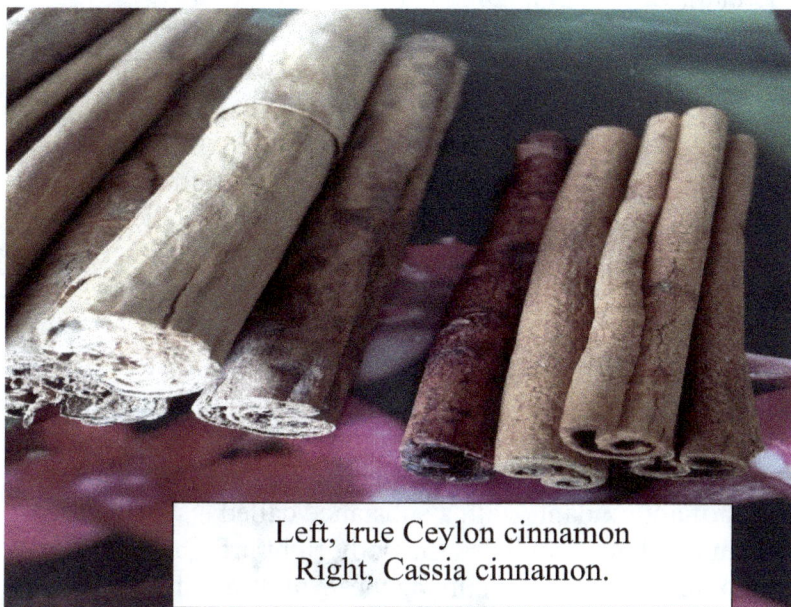

Left, true Ceylon cinnamon
Right, Cassia cinnamon.

**Cinnamon**

Cinnamon has been used by humans for thousands of years, noted by its mention in the Old Testament for its benefits as an anointing and perfuming oil.

The four basic commercially available types are Ceylon Cinnamon, Cassia or Chinese Cinnamon, Saigon Cinnamon, and Korintje Cinnamon. Chinese Cinnamon, mostly produced in Indonesia, is the primary cinnamon found in North America, and Ceylon cinnamon, produced in Sri Lanka, the most widely used in Europe. The purest form with strongest healing ingredients is the Ceylon cinnamon (Cinnamomum zeyanicium). I prefer this one over the cassia types produced in Indonesia, China, and Vietnam. Ceylon cinnamon is light brown, easily distinguished from the cassia type whose color is muddy brown. If you buy cinnamon sticks, you will find that cassia sticks are very hard and are tucked in the form of a hollow tube. Because of their density, they're especially difficult to grind. Genuine Ceylon sticks are thin and brittle, easily broken, and the inside has a full-bodied, cigarette-like appearance. See the photo that demonstrates the difference.

The benefits of cinnamon are numerous. For example, it's antioxidant properties protect the body from many diseases. Cinnamon boosts the immune system and has an antibacterial effect. Cinnamon even surpasses garlic in terms of antioxidants with a substance called cinnamaldehyde that helps the body fight inflammation. Cinnamon is rich in iron, manganese, and calcium. To help prevent and treat colds, mix one tablespoon of honey with a quarter teaspoon of cinnamon powder and swallow daily. You can swirl the mixture into green or black tea.

Be sure you use genuine cinnamon, as some cassia has been reported to cause liver damage. Cinnamon should be taken in moderation, with one teaspoon the daily recommended amount.

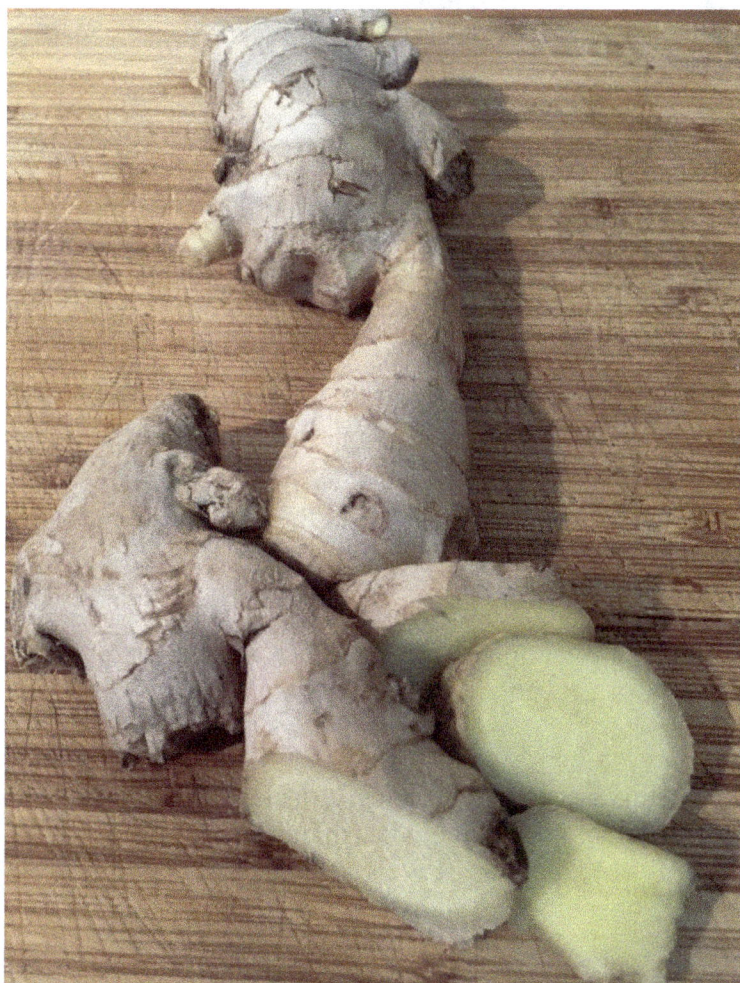

**Ginger.** (Zingiber officinale). Ginger is in the family Zingiberaceae. It's an herbaceous perennial that grows around stems about a meter tall bearing narrow green leaves and yellow flowers. Both the spicy leaves and the ginger root have been used as a natural medicine for more than 2000 years. Most of the commercial ginger comes from China.

Both fresh roots and finely dried ground can be found on the shelves of the ginger shop. Ginger stimulates the body to remove toxins and cleanses the lymphatic system. Its antioxidants kill a variety of bacteria and inhibit inflammation. It is useful for prophylactic use by adding to dishes or teas.

It's better not to pour pieces of ginger root into boiling soup or sauce, because at high temperatures ginger loses its good properties. So, if you make ginger tea with honey, pour everything in boiled water that's allowed to cool.

**Ginger Health Benefits**

1. Heart Protection. It reduces blood clotting and can serve as a preventive measure against stroke and heart attacks.

2. Aid for Digestion. It helps to relieve constipation. In the morning, put a slice of cut ginger in a cup of boiled water, cover the cup, leave for 10-15 minutes (until the ginger is absorbed) and drink.

3. Flu Prevention. Add some sliced ginger to a cup of boiled water. After allowing the mixture to cool, add pressed lemon juice and a teaspoon of honey.

4. Immunity Enhancement. Ayurvedic medicine recommends using ginger as a spice to strengthen the immune system.

5. Prevention of cancer. Ginger fights against aggressive and severe forms of lung, colon, breast, prostate, and ovarian cancer.

6. Prevention of diabetes. Studies have shown that ginger can contribute to healing diabetes. Ginger reduces the sugar content in the blood, as well as excess fat and cholesterol.

7. Menstrual pains. Ginger can help young women suffering from menstrual pains.

8. Ginger stimulates the body to remove toxins and cleanses the lymphatic system.

9. Antioxidant. Ginger kills a variety of bacteria and inhibits inflammation.

**Warnings about the use of ginger:** It can interact with many medications, such as anti-inflammatory drugs, heart pills, and blood thinners. Ginger can cause allergies during pregnancy, and worsen certain illnesses, such as gallbladder stones, stomach ulcers, herpes, and acne. Ginger suppresses the absorption of iron and fat-soluble vitamins. Due to blood thinning effects, it shouldn't be used within two weeks of anticipated surgery.

Fresh ginger is commonly used for teas, but it is possible to add some ginger to a variety of beverages and cocktails. Ginger powder can be used as a spice for burgers or salad.

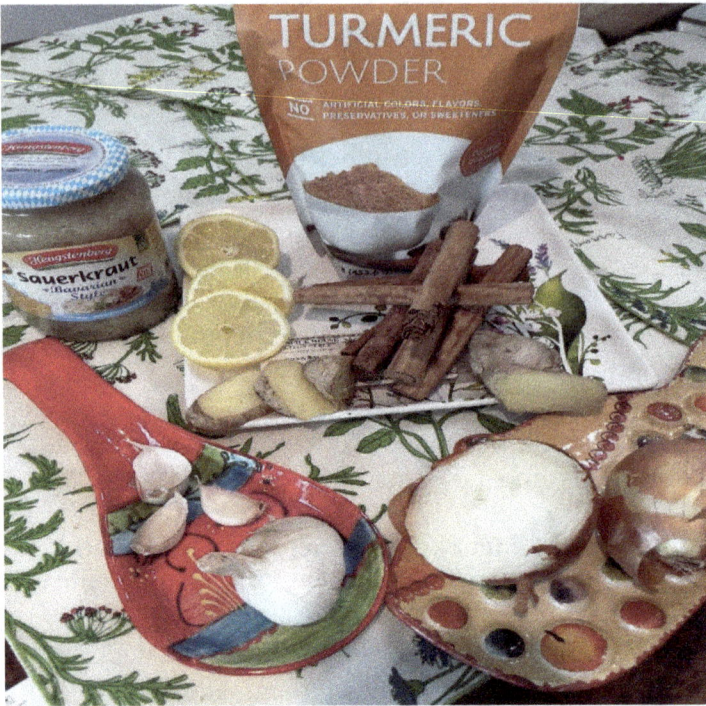

**Turmeric** (Curcuma longa). Turmeric is a perennial plant of the Zingiberaceae ginger family and is a species of the Curcuma ginger family. This spice is widely used in Indian, Middle Eastern, South American, and Asian cuisines.

It can grow up to 90 cm in height, with large simple leaves. The flower blossoms with green on the bottom and white on the top. There are small tubes in their yellow blossoms. Turmeric supplements come from the plant's rhizomes, which feature rough, brown skin and a dark orange flesh, and are available in liquid extract, capsule, and powder forms.

Commonly used in Asian food, you probably know turmeric as the main spice in curry, giving it a distinctive flavor and yellow color. The root of turmeric is also used widely to make medicine.

Turmeric is rich in vitamins C, A, B1, B2, B3, and E, as well as micro elements such as iron, calcium, phosphorus, iodine. Turmeric has antiviral, antifungal, anti-inflammatory, and anti-carcinogenic properties. Due to its antioxidant properties, it helps to remove free radicals from the body.

The main use for turmeric is to reduce inflammation such as suppressing arthritis pain, joint inflammation, muscle pain, and to relief other chronic inflammatory pains. Due to its antioxidant properties, turmeric is suitable for the treatment of liver diseases.

Other traditional uses include regulating gastrointestinal activity and improving digestion, dissolving fatty meals, antibiotic properties, prediabetic and diabetic supplements, treatment of skin ulcers and prostate cancer, reduction of cholesterol levels, treating cold symptoms, strengthening the immune system, encouraging wound healing, and weight control. Turmeric tea, high with antioxidants, helps prevent Alzheimer's disease, and can be used as an antiseptic ointment in skincare. In Indian medicine, turmeric is used for the treatment of itching, dermatitis, and allergic rash. They create a paste containing the turmeric and apply it directly to the diseased skin, such as ulcers, eczema, and infected sites.

The food naturalist, B. Baratinskaite, suggests using a pinch of turmeric to flavor omelets, soups, salads, rice, legumes, and cabbage dishes.

**Dosage:** 500 mg of curcumin per day.

**Do not use turmeric** to treat bile duct obstruction or if you have bile duct stones. Turmeric should not be used in the treatment of infertility or for the treatment of blood disorders. Large turmeric levels inhibit blood clotting and should not be used if you have gastric ulcers, increased acidity in your stomach, pancreatitis. Don't use turmeric if you are pregnant or an infant-feeding mother, or if you have immune system disorders or allergic symptoms.

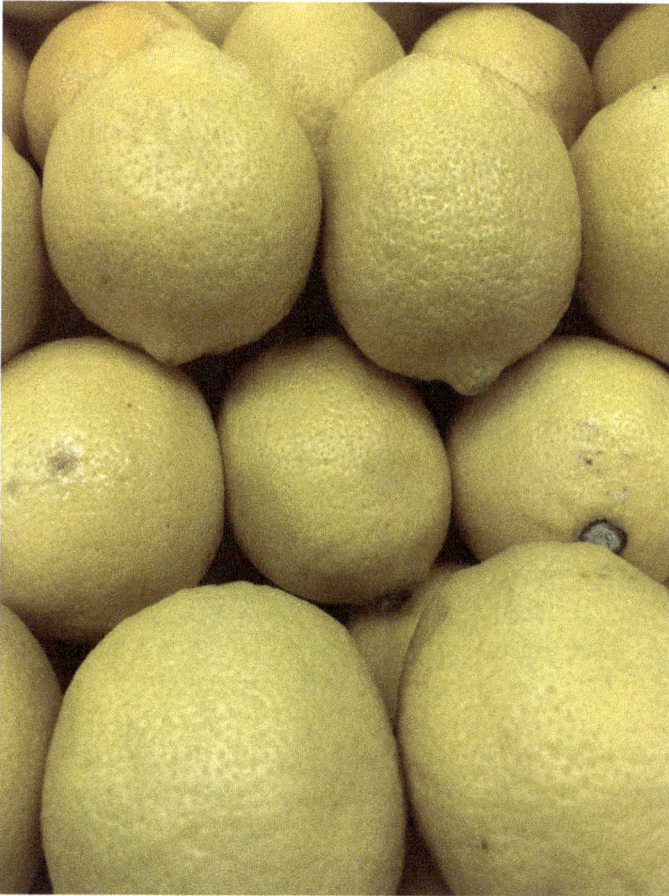

**Lemon** (Citrus: Limon). It is believed that lemons originated from the Himalayan Mountains located in the east of India and then spread around the world, growing best in temperate and tropical climates. The lime (or green lemon) is smaller than the lemon and less sour. The lemon is one of the most widely used fruits in the world.

Sailors and researchers began using lemons in the 18th century, where they had to spend a long time on board without fresh fruit and vegetables. At that time, sailors often suffered from scurvy (vitamin C deficiency), sight disorders, gum bleeding, and teeth falling out. In 1747, Scott James Lind established that lemons and oranges could help avoid scurvy and treat it. By the end of the 18th century, English navy had declared that every sailor had to drink 30ml of lemon juice daily. Nowadays, lemons are used for flavoring teas, salad dressings, garnishes, marinades, desserts, and drinks.

**Health Benefits of Lemons**

Vitamin C, a powerful antioxidant found in lemon juice, neutralizes free radicals and protects against cancer. Lemons have antimicrobial effects against bacterial and fungal infections. They are also effective against parasites and worms and regulate blood pressure if it is too high. The lemon is an antidepressant and helps those struggling with stress and nervous disorders.

Vitamin C is extremely important for maintaining the immune system, producing white blood cells, and delaying premature aging. Vitamin C plays an important role in collagen production, which is responsible for skin elasticity and improving skin structure. Eating foods that contain high levels of vitamin C and iron will maximize iron absorption to prevent and treat anemia.

To live a healthy life, you can start each morning with a glass of warm water squeezed with fresh lemon juice. Such a drink not only strengthens the immune system, but also helps to regulate the acidity of the body, because lemons are rich in alkaline substances, which reduce acidity. These alkaline properties work best when lemon juice is diluted with water. The use of shaved lemon peel in cooking is also recommended, as the peel is rich in essential oils with antiviral and antiseptic properties – preventing viruses and colds.

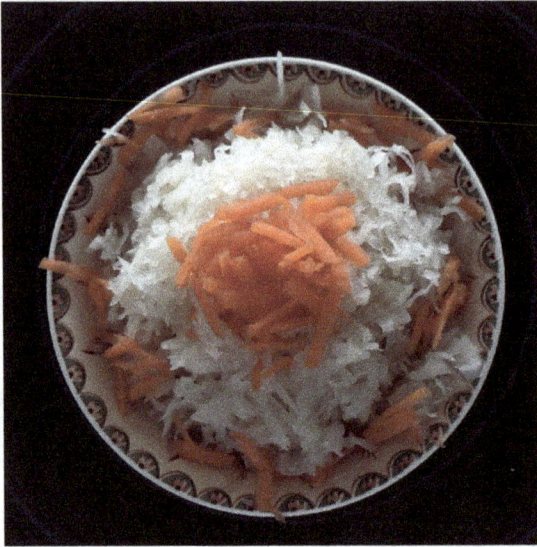

## Sauerkraut

Sauerkraut is finely cut raw cabbage (Brassica oleracea) that has been fermented by lactic acid producing bacteria. It has a long shelf life and a distinctive sour flavor, both of which result from the lactic acid formed when the bacteria ferment the sugars in cabbage leaves. It is one of the best-known national dishes in Germany and throughout Eastern Europe. In the Netherlands it is known as zuurkool, in France, choucroute. The English name is borrowed from Germany where it means "sour cabbage." Sauerkraut, like other preserved foods, provided a source of nutrients during the winter. Captain James Cook always took a store of sauerkraut on this sea voyage to prevent scurvy. Chopped cabbage is often pickled together with other ingredients for addition flavor, such as shredded carrots. caraway seeds, whole or quartered apples, and cranberry.

**Health Benefits of Sauerkraut**

Cabbage is a very strong antioxidant that neutralizes the effects of aggressive radicals. These abundant antioxidants not only prevent breast cancer, but also the formation of malignant tumors in other organs, notably the lungs, the bladder, the large intestine, and the stomach. Cabbage can help certain kinds of headaches, but only consuming it, not by putting a cabbage leaf on your forehead.

Sauerkraut contains fiber, carbs, calcium, iron, zinc, potassium, and vitamins A, K, C, B-6, and folate. Vitamin B-6 improves digestive activity. The acid in cabbage cleanses the intestines and removes toxins. The trace elements in cabbage improve energy and help to strengthen immunity. Sauerkraut's vitamins strengthen the heart muscle and help normalize blood sugar and cholesterol. Folate helps fight depression. Magnesium-can help regulate blood pressure.

According to nutrition expert B. Baratinskaite, "In order to meet the daily requirements of vitamin C, one need eat about 300grams of sauerkraut (about 10 oz)."

**When cabbage is not recommended.**

Sauerkraut is not healthy for patients with stomach ulcers, gastritis, or pancreatitis. Sauerkraut is harmful in people with kidney and liver diseases because the dish contains a large amount of salt. To lower the salt content, rinse cabbage with water before preparing the meal.

When shopping for sauerkraut, look for the unpasteurized product that does not have vinegar. When heat is used for pasteurization, the beneficial bacteria are often destroyed. The label should state that there are live active cultures. Remember to look for sugar content as well. Too much sugar just adds unneeded sweetness and calories.

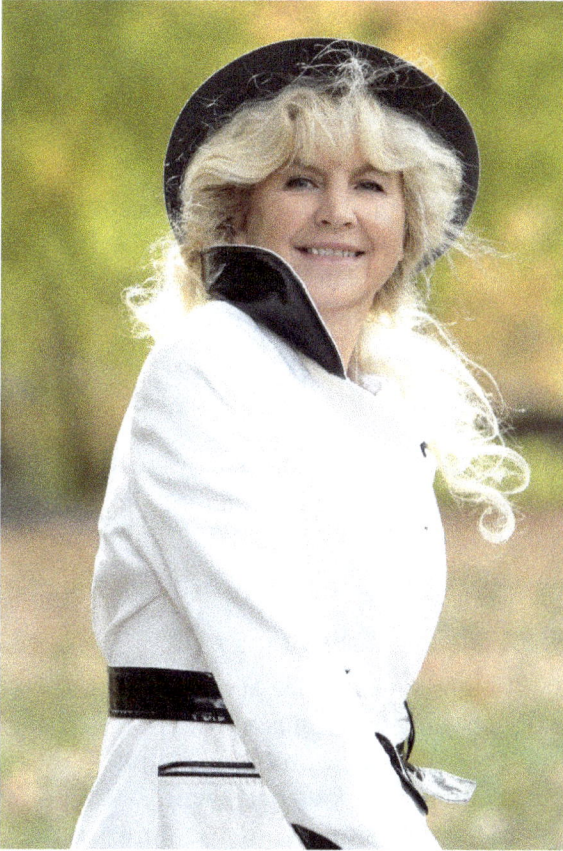

## Other Ways to Stay Healthy

Although this book is primarily about the value of grains in your diet, as well as a few special foods just listed, it's important to remember other important aspects of a healthy life.

**The Power of Salt Water**

Ancient Egyptians took health very seriously, claiming to be the healthiest people in the world after Libyans. They practiced cleanliness rituals. Because soap was still unknown, they used ashes or soda which are both good detergents and dissolve fatty matter. They used salt water for healing purposes. Frescoes in ancient Egyptian pyramids have depictions of pharaohs using salt after a hot bath, with their whole bodies wrapped in salted parchment as they climb into a hot bath.

Ukrainian chemist professor B. Bolotov explains, "If the activity of lymph nodes is weakened, the body can't fight cancer cells, bacteria, viruses, or fungi. Bathing in salt water invigorates these nodes." He advises a hot bath to treat joint diseases.

To make your salt bath: soak 1-2 kg of salt in a normal-size 30-gallon bathtub, soaking 1-2 times a week for 15-20 minutes. If you do not have a bathtub, take a hot shower for 2-3 minutes, and then rub your body with salt for a few minutes, enough to turn the skin red. Rinse lightly with warm water so that you feel a slight saltiness afterwards.

**Regular Exercise:**

In order to strengthen the body's resistance to infectious organisms, it is very important to be physically active. Exercises, such as rapid walks or dancing, improves the functioning of the circulatory and lymphatic systems. When a person lives a passive life, immunity is weakened.

## Spiritual Health

In order to be healthy, it is important to develop not only the body, but also spiritual qualities. Spiritual qualities have a great influence on human life, such as forgiveness, kindness, love, pleasure, bliss, reconciliation, charm, wonder, spiritual upliftment, joy, and faith. Spiritual health will help you overcome obstacles, difficulties, and sometimes serious illnesses. Gloomy, dark emotions produce poison, complicating the functioning of various organs and functions. Bright emotions improve the functioning of all body functions and activate the production of serotonin, the happiness hormone.

Resistance to disease is also greatly enhanced by saunas, walks in nature, breathing fresh air, meditation, massages, and aroma therapy.

## Glossary

**Ancient:** Refers to anything considered very old.

**Allergy:** Allergic diseases are a number of conditions caused by hypersensitivity of the immune system to typically harmless substances in the environment.

**Alzheimer:** Chronic neurodegenerative disease that usually starts and worsens over time. A progressive form of dementia.

**Antibacterial:** Anything that destroys bacteria or suppresses their growth.

**Antibiotics:** A type of antimicrobial substance active against bacteria used to fight bacterial infections.

**Antioxidants:** Found in many foods, including fruits and vegetables. They are also available as dietary supplements.

**Antiseptic:** A substance that stops or slows down the growth of microorganisms.

**Aromatherapy:** Uses plant materials and aromatic plant oils, including essential oils and other aroma compounds for improving psychological or physical well-being.

**Asafetida:** A fetid resinous gum obtained from the roots of an herbaceous plant, used in herbal medicine and Indian cooking.

**Aztecs:** A member of the indigenous people dominant in Mexico before the Spanish conquest of the 16th century.

**Baking soda:** A natural mineral (Sodium Bicarbonate).

**Beta-glucans:** Comprise a group of B-D-glucose polysaccharides naturally occurring in the walls of cereal, bacteria, and fungi with significant physicochemical properties dependent on source.

**Cancer:** A malignant tumor.

**Carbohydrates:** The most widespread organic substances. They play a vital role in all life.

**Cardiac:** Relating to the heart.

**Celiac disease:** A digestive problem that damages the small intestine and interferes with the absorption of nutrients.

**Cholesterol:** Fat-like material in blood and most tissues.

**Collagen:** The main structural protein in the extracellular space in the various connective tissues in animal bodies.

**Dal:** Often known as lentils, but actually refers to a split version of a number of lentils, peas, chickpeas, kidney beans etc. If lentils are split into half, they're called dal.

**Depressant:** Reduces nervous or functional activity.

**Diabetes:** A disorder of the metabolism causing excessive thirst and the production of large volumes of urine. Most commonly diabetes mellitus, inefficient sugar management resulting in excess body sugar.

**E-100:** Food coloring agent as a yellow pigment.

**Flavonoids:** A group of plant metabolites thought to provide health benefits through cell signaling pathways and antioxidant effects.

**Fungus:** A member of the group of eukaryotic organisms that includes microorganisms such as yeasts and molds, as well as the more familiar mushrooms.

**Gelatin:** An animal protein mixture.

**Gluten:** A protein food in grains.

**Gluten-Free Diet:** An eating plan that excludes foods containing gluten.

**GMO:** Genetically modified organisms.

**Hypertension:** High blood pressure.

**Hippocrates:** Known as the "Father of Medicine," c460–c377 BC. Greek physician.

**Immune system:** The body's protective system which provides antibodies to defend against infection and diseases.

**Lymphatic system:** The tissues and organs that produce, store, and carry white blood cells that fight infections and other diseases.

**Matzah:** A thin unleavened bread made from flour and water that's traditionally eaten during Passover.

**Mayan:** A member of an American Indian people of Yucatan and Belize and Guatemala who had a culture that reached its peak between AD 300 and 900, characterized by outstanding architecture and pottery and astronomy. Mayans had a system of writing and an accurate calendar.

**Metabolism:** The chemical processes that occur within a living organism in order to maintain life.

**Microbes:** A microorganism, especially a bacterium causing disease.

**Nutrients:** A substance that provides nourishment essential for growth and the maintenance of life.

**Ras El Hanout:** Moroccan spice blend.

**Phytochemicals:** Compounds that are produced by plants ("Phyto" means "plant"). They are found in fruits, vegetables, grains, beans, and other plants. Some of these phytochemicals are believed to protect cells from damage that could lead to cancer.

**Processed food:** Any food that has been altered in some way during preparation.

**Sauna:** A small room used as a hot-air or steam bath for cleaning and refreshing the body.

**Scurvy:** A disease resulting from a lack of vitamins.

**Serotonin:** The happiness hormone.

**Thrombi:** A blood clot formed in situ within the vascular system of the body and impeding blood flow.

**King Tut's name meaning:** King Tut was born circa 1341 BCE in ancient Egypt. He was given the name Tutankhaten, meaning "The living image of Aten." After taking power, the boy king changed his name to Tutankhamun, which means "The living image of Amun."

**Vigor:** Physical strength and good health.

## Plant Name and Other Important Subject Index

**Bold** type indicates plant warning, other side effects.

## Subject Index

blood circulation 39
blood clots 38, 77
blood sugar 30, 34, 39, 51, 86
body cleansers 70
blood sugar 30, 34, 39, 51, 86
blood thinning 78
blood vessels 38, 39
blood pressure 34, 38, 39, 40, 65, 70, 83

**C**
calcium 19,46, 61, 73, 75, 80, 86
cancer  34, 40, 60, 61, 70, 77, 80, 83, 86
carbohydrates 16, 26, 27, 32, 60, 86
cardiovascular 34, 39, 51, 65, 70
carotenoids 71
celiac disease 17, 25, 27, 29, 60
chia seeds 23, 64, 67
cholesterol reducers 34, 38, 39, 40, 51, 60, 65, 80, 86
cinnamon 74
  cinnamaldehide 75
collagen 51, 83
cold 75, 80, 84
constipation 77
copper 51
cosmetics 29, 45

**D**
depression 86
dermatitis 80
diabetes 51, 60, 61, 78
  supplements 80
digestion 77, 80
digestive 17, 40, 60
duodenal ulcer 73
eczema 81
energy boosters 16, 23, 30, 34, 38, 39, 65, 86
enzymes 71

**F**

fatigue 27, 70
fibers 16, 17, 18, 19, 27
  dietary 34, 39, 40, 46, 65
flavonoids 19
flu prevention 70, 77
folate 65, 86
folic acid 38
fungi 73

## G
gallbladder 78
gas 17
gastrointestinal diseases 27, 34, 51
gastritis 86
genetic manipulation 17
gluten 17, 20, 25, 26, 27, 46
  intolerance 27, 29
gluten-free 19, 20, 23, 25, 27, 29, 51, 60
GMO 65

## H
headaches 86
healthy benefits 34, 90
heart 60, 61, 77
herpes 78

## I
immune system 34, 51, 68, 70, 77, 80 84, 86, 89
  response 25, 75, 83
inflammation 60, 75, 70, 77, 80
infections 83
insulin 30, 39
inulin 71
intestines 70, 86
  parasites 70
iodine 80
iron 20, 38, 46, 60, 65, 75, 80, 86
  absorption 78

## L

lactic acid 85
lemon peels 84
live cultures 87
liver damage75
longevity 7, 8, 11, 12, 13, 88, 89, 90
lymphatic system 77, 78

## M

magnesium 51, 65, 86
malignant tumors 86
massages 90
manganese 18, 19, 51, 65, 75
meditation 90
menstrual pain 78
microbes 19, 20, 34, 38, 65
microelements 71
minerals 16, 17, 18, 20, 32, 34, 38, 39, 45, 60
mood 70

## N

nervous disorders 83
nutritious 16, 17, 19, 20, 23, 24, 27, 28, 38, 40, 46, 51, 85
  diet 29
nutty flavor 19

## O

Omega-3 fatty acids 20, 65
oxidative 40

## P

pancreas 39
pancreatitis 86
parasites 83
pectin 71
phenolic acids 19
phosphorus 51, 60, 65, 80
phytochemicals 60
pollen 24

potassium 20, 38, 39, 86
prediabetic supplement 80
processed food 21
pseudo cereal 24

**R**
radioactive isotopes 38
rashes 27, 80
riboflavin 65
rutin 39

**S**
salt 86, 87, 89
saturated fat 46
saunas 83
sensitivity 27
silicon 51
skin care 70, 80, 81, 83
  ulcers 80
  itching 80
spiritual qualities 90
stress 83
starchy 19. 51
stomach ulcers 78, 86
stroke 77
sugar 46, 60, 87

**T**
thiamine 18, 65
toxins 86

**V**
vinegar 87
viruses 70, 84
vitamins 16, 17, 18, 20, 32, 60
  A 80, 86
  B 20, 34, 38, 45, 46, 65
  B1 16, 71, 80
  B2 16, 71, 80

102

B3 80
B6 86
C 20, 71, 80, 83, 86
E 16, 46, 80
K 86
PP 16, 71

**W**
water retention 17
wheat 17
  free 20, 29
  modern 17, 20, 21
  sensitivity 60
weight 27, 29, 32, 60, 80
worms 83
wound healing 80

**Z**
zinc 60, 65, 85

## FOOD RECIPES and PREPARATIONS

## Bibliography

Paul Bragg, **Healthy Lifestyle**, Publisher Health
   Science1999.
Michel Genest and Dan Jason, **Awesome Ancient
   Grains and seeds: A Garden -To-Kitchen Guide**,
   Publisher Douglas and McIntyre 2013.
Regina Nedas **The Therapy of Natural Living,**
   Publishing by Doctor's Dreams Publishing United
   States of America  2019.
Joseph Murray, **Mayo Clinic Going Gluten Free**,
   Publishing Time Inc., Books 2014.
Peter H. R. Green and Rory Jones, **Celiac Disease: A
   Hidden epidemic**, Publishing HarperCollins 2016.
Case Adams, and **The Gluten Cure: Scientifically
   Proven Natural Solutions to Celiac Disease
   Gluten Sensitivities**, Publishing Logical Books
   2014.
Maria Speck, **Ancient Grains for Modern Meals**,
   Publisher Potter/Ten Speed/Harmony Rodale 2011.
Ross A.Laird, **Grain Of Truth: The Ancient Lessons
   of Craft**, Publisher Walker and Company 2002.
Ann Taylor Pittman, **Everyday Whole Grains: 175
   New Recipes From Amaranth to Wild Rice,
   Including Every Ancient Grain,** Publisher Time
   Inc., Books 2016.
Maria Speck, **Simply Ancient Grains: Fresh and
   Flavorful Whole Grain Recipes for Living Well**,
   Publisher Potter/Ten Speed/Harmony Rodale 2015.
Najmieh Batmanglij, **Food of Life**: Ancient Persian and
   Modern Iranian cooking and Ceremonies, Mage
   Publishers INC, Washington DC 2020.

Stephen Yafa, **Grain Of Truth: The Real Case for and Against Wheat and Gluten**, Penguin Publishing Group 2015.

Patricia Green and Carolyn Hemming, **Grain Power: Over 100 Delicious Gluten-Free Ancient Grain and Superblend Recipes**, Publisher Penguin Canada 2014.

Maria Baez Kijac, **Cooking with Ancient Grains**, Publisher Adams Media Corporation 2014.

Laura B Mc, **Bridge Cooking with Ancient Grains**, Create Space independent Publishing Platform 2013.

B. Bolotov, G. Pogozhev, **Narodnyy Lechebnik Bolotova**, Publisher Piter SPb, Russia 2013.

Author's Team, **Everything With Buckwheat,** Lithuania, 1987.

Patricia Green, Carolyn Hemming, **Quinoa: The Everyday Super Food 365**, Canada 2011.

Lauri Boane, **Superfood For Life, Chia**, Published Fair Winds Press 2014.

Danna Washburn and Heather Butt, **The Gluten-Free Baking**, Published by Robert Rose Inc. Canada 2011.

Author's Team, **Russian, Polish and German Cooking**, Annes Publishing LTD London, 2007, 2008.

**Internet**

Bruno Ferrero,**Two Seeds,** thoughts.lt, (mintys.lt) Lithuania 2011.

Swasthi, **How to cook millet by Swasthi,** June 3, 2020.

Shalini Rajani, **Buckwheat,** The Indian Express 2021.

Shalini Rajani, **Harness the power of buckwheat with this scrumptious salad**, The Indian Express, 2020.

Everything you need to know about the most popular
grains, **Cook Book.lt** (Virtuves Knyga.lt) Lithuania
2011.
Jolinda Hackett, **What are Ancient Grains - The
Spruce Eats**, 2019.

**Magazines**
BBC News Magazine's by Joanna Jolly, **Why Do
American Love Ancient Grains**, 12/15/2014.

**Newspapers**
Arunas Jonuskis, **The Power of Salt Water**, Peasant
Newspaper Lithuania 2021/02/25.

**Bulletin**
AARP **Live Longer, Stronger Better**, Published May
2021.

www.ingramcontent.com/pod-product-compliance
Lightning Source LLC
Chambersburg PA
CBHW052051270326
41931CB00012B/2712